Endocrine Diseases in Pregnancy and the Postpartum Period

Endocrine Diseases in Pregnancy and the Postpartum Period

Edited by

Nadia Barghouthi, MD, MPH

Assistant Professor, Department of Medicine
Section of Endocrinology & Metabolism

and

Assistant Program Director
West Virginia University Endocrinology Fellowship
West Virginia University
Morgantown, West Virginia

Jessica Perini, MD, MS

Associate Professor, Department of Medicine
Section of Endocrinology & Metabolism

and

Interim Division Chief, Endocrinology Program Director
West Virginia University Endocrinology Fellowship
West Virginia University
Morgantown, West Virginia

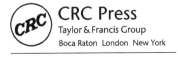

CRC Press
Taylor & Francis Group
Boca Raton London New York

CRC Press is an imprint of the
Taylor & Francis Group, an **informa** business

First edition published 2022
by CRC Press
6000 Broken Sound Parkway NW, Suite 300, Boca Raton, FL 33487-2742

and by CRC Press
2 Park Square, Milton Park, Abingdon, Oxon, OX14 4RN

© 2022 Taylor & Francis Group, LLC

CRC Press is an imprint of Taylor & Francis Group, LLC

Library of Congress Cataloging-in-Publication Data

Names: Barghouthi, Nadia, editor. | Perini, Jessica, MD, editor.
Title: Endocrine diseases in pregnancy and the postpartum period / edited by Nadia Barghouthi, Jessica Perini.
Description: First edition. | Boca Raton, FL; Abingdon, Oxon: CRC Press /Taylor & Francis Group, 2022. | Includes bibliographical references and index. | Summary: "This book delivers comprehensive explanations of normal hormonal physiology during pregnancy and descriptions of the hormonal pathology associated with various endocrine disease states. Evaluation and management of endocrine disorders including but not limited to diabetes mellitus, thyroid disease, and various endocrine tumors are included"—Provided by publisher.
Identifiers: LCCN 2021049578 (print) | LCCN 2021049579 (ebook) | ISBN 9780367462178 (paperback) | ISBN 9781032198354 (hardback) | ISBN 9781003027577 (ebook)
Subjects: MESH: Endocrine System Diseases—complications | Pregnancy Complications—physiopathology | Postpartum Period
Classification: LCC RG811 (print) | LCC RG811 (ebook) | NLM WK 140 | DDC 618.7/4—dc23/eng/20211101
LC record available at https://lccn.loc.gov/2021049578
LC ebook record available at https://lccn.loc.gov/2021049579

ISBN: 978-1-032-19835-4 (hbk)
ISBN: 978-0-367-46217-8 (pbk)
ISBN: 978-1-003-02757-7 (ebk)

DOI: 10.1201/9781003027577

Typeset in Minion
by KnowledgeWorks Global Ltd.

Dedication

To my heart, Luca, and my love, Brandon. To my father, mother, and sister who always inspire me.

Nadia Barghouthi

To my children, Alessandro, Rafael, and Natalia who are the lights of my life and to my husband, Ivan, who provides constant love and support. And Kiki.

Jessica Perini

To all of our family, friends, and colleagues who continue to love, support, and motivate us.

Contents

Preface

We are happy to present our book, *Endocrine Diseases in Pregnancy and the Postpartum Period.* Our goal in writing and compiling this work is to provide an endocrine manual that is comprehensive and easy to use. All major endocrine topics that students, residents, and all providers of healthcare may face when working with pregnant patients are included. From evaluating hyperglycemia in the prenatal period to managing thyroid storm in pregnancy, the book aims to cover diagnosis, evaluation, and management of the multitude of endocrine disorders. Many of the topics discussed apply to nonpregnant patients as well. We have opted to organize the information in bullet point form for ease of use and reference.

As two endocrinologists who love our chosen specialty, we know that endocrinology can sometimes seem obscure. Our plan with this book is to make endocrinology accessible and management of endocrine disorders straightforward. We are confident that this book will become a well-thumbed pocket manual for all things endocrine.

Nadia Barghouthi, MD MPH
Jessica Perini, MD MS

Acknowledgments

We would like to acknowledge our favorite historian, Brandon R. Roos, for all of his assistance in editing, source formatting, and proofreading. We thank him for allowing us to use his expertise in writing and academic research to help this book come to fruition.

Editors

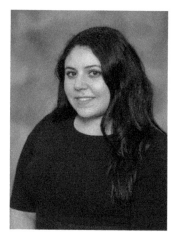

Nadia Barghouthi, MD, MPH, is an endocrinologist and Assistant Professor at West Virginia University. She serves as the Assistant Program Director of the West Virginia University School of Medicine Endocrinology Fellowship. A long-time resident of the Mountain State and a lifelong WVU Mountaineer, Dr. Barghouthi is passionate about educating the next generation of clinicians and researchers and has used her position to advocate for disadvantaged and underserved communities within the healthcare system. Her academic research has included studies on diabetes mellitus and pheochromocytomas. An avid teacher, she greatly enjoys lecturing medical students, residents, and fellows on a wide range of endocrine topics and is always ready to help students achieve their individual academic and professional goals. She serves on several committees within the university related to inpatient diabetes management, academic standards and core competencies, quality improvement, and transgender health. Her clinical interests include adrenal disorders and neuroendocrine tumors.

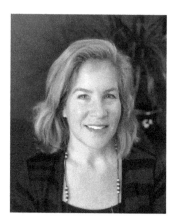

Jessica Perini, MD, MS, is an endocrinologist and Associate Professor at West Virginia University. She serves as the Program Director of the West Virginia University School of Medicine Endocrinology Fellowship. She also serves as the interim Section Chair of the WVU Endocrinology Division. Teaching is one of her many passions and she enjoys mentoring future endocrinologists through the American Association of Clinical Endocrinology (AACE)-sponsored programs such as their web-based mentorship program and Endocrine University. Dr. Perini has engaged in research ranging from cystic fibrosis, diabetes mellitus, and osteoporosis. She serves as an elected member of the WVU Internal Medicine Advisory Committee and holds leadership positions on a number of other committees within the WVU School of Medicine. In her own practice, she is particularly interested in supporting the care of the transgender population of Appalachia and improving the quality of care for underserved populations within West Virginia.

Contributors

Vivek Alaigh MD
Stamford Health Medical Group
Stamford, Connecticut

Dushyanthy Arasaratnam MD
Department of Endocrinology
Mount Sinai Beth Israel
New York, New York

Vladimer Bakhutashvili MD
Department of Endocrinology
University of Virginia
Charlottesville, Virginia

Ela Banerjee MD
Department of Endocrinology
Brown University Warren Alpert Medical School
Providence, Rhode Island

Nadia Barghouthi MD, MPH
Department of Medicine
Section of Endocrinology & Metabolism
and
West Virginia University Endocrinology Fellowship
West Virginia University
Morgantown, West Virginia

Harikrashna Bhatt MD
Endocrinology
Brown University Warren Alpert Medical School
and
Providence VA Medical Center
Providence, Rhode Island

Vicky Cheng MD
Endocrinology
Brown University Warren Alpert Medical School
Providence, Rhode Island

Fiona J. Cook MD
Division of Endocrinology
East Carolina University
Greenville, North Carolina

Loren Custer MD
Department of Obstetrics & Gynecology
West Virginia University
Morgantown, West Virginia

Laura Davisson MD, MPH
Department of Medicine
WVU Medicine Medical and Surgical Weight Loss
    Center
West Virginia University
Morgantown, West Virginia

Sejal Doshi MD
Department of Endocrinology
Brown University Warren Alpert Medical School
Providence, Rhode Island

Rawan El-Amin DO, MPH
Department of Obstetrics & Gynecology
West Virginia University
Morgantown, West Virginia

Shira B. Eytan MD
Department of Medicine
Park Avenue Endocrinology and Nutrition
New York University Grossman School of
    Medicine
New York, New York

Krystel Feghali MD
Department of Endocrinology
Baystate Medical Center
Springfield, Massachusetts

Amanda Fernandes MD
Endocrinology
Brown University Warren Alpert Medical
    School
Providence, Rhode Island

Valerie B. Galvan Turner MD
Gynecologic Oncology Department of Women's
    Health
Dell Medical School
University of Texas
Austin, Texas

Jennifer Giordano DO
Department of Medicine
Section of Endocrinology & Metabolism
West Virginia University
Morgantown, West Virginia

Adnan Haider MD
Department of Medicine
Section of Endocrinology & Metabolism
West Virginia University
Morgantown, West Virginia

Gayatri Jaiswal MD
Center for Diabetes and Endocrine Health
Allegheny Health Network
Pittsburgh, Pennsylvania

Maria Javaid MD
Department of Medicine
Section of Endocrinology, Diabetes, and
    Metabolism
and
Diabetes and Endocrinology Center
Shalamar Institute of Health Sciences
Lahore, Pakistan

Maitri Shelly Kalia-Reynolds DO, MS
Endocrinology
Blanchard Valley Health System
Findlay, Ohio

Julia C.W. Lake MD
Department of Endocrinology
Dartmouth Hitchcock Medical Center
Lebanon, New Hampshire

Jasmin Lebastchi MD
Endocrinology
Brown University Warren Alpert Medical School
Providence, Rhode Island

Anthony Parravani MD
Department of Medicine
Section of Nephrology
West Virginia University
Morgantown, West Virginia

Bethany Pellegrino MD
Department of Medicine
Section of Nephrology
West Virginia University
Morgantown, West Virginia

Jessica Perini MD, MS
Department of Medicine
Section of Endocrinology & Metabolism
and
West Virginia University Endocrinology Fellowship
West Virginia University
Morgantown, West Virginia

Reshmitha Radhakrishnan MD
Internal Medicine
Brown University Warren Alpert Medical School
Providence, Rhode Island

Tharani Rajeswaran MD
Endocrinology
Brown University Warren Alpert Medical School
Providence, Rhode Island

Beatriz Francesca Ramirez MD
Department of Endocrinology
VMC Medical Director Inpatient Diabetes Program
Brody School of Medicine
East Carolina University
Greenville, North Carolina

Rashi Sandooja MD
Department of Endocrinology, Diabetes, and
    Nutrition
Mayo Clinic
Rochester, Minnesota

Rohma Shamsi MD
Department of Medicine
Section of Endocrinology & Metabolism
West Virginia University
Morgantown, West Virginia

Jennifer Silk DO
Department of Obstetrics & Gynecology
West Virginia University
Morgantown, West Virginia

Jeremy Soule MD
Physicians of Charleston
West Virginia University School of Medicine,
 Charleston Campus
Charleston, West Virginia

Oksana Symczyk MD
Department of Medicine
Section of Endocrinology & Metabolism
West Virginia University
Morgantown, West Virginia

Jennifer S. Turner MD
Department of Medicine
Section of Endocrinology & Metabolism
West Virginia University
Morgantown, West Virginia

Robert Weingold MD
Department of Endocrinology
Yale University
New Haven, Connecticut

CHAPTER 1

Physiology of Pregnancy and Lactation

Normal physiology of pregnancy

RAWAN EL-AMIN, LOREN CUSTER, AND JENNIFER SILK

KEY POINTS

- Pregnancy induces a state of physiologic water and sodium retention, largely regulated by the posterior pituitary and renin-angiotensin-aldosterone system (RAAS). An increase in glomerular filtration rate (GFR) alters the excretion of electrolytes and nutrients.
- Blood pressure, cardiac output, and cardiac structure are altered during pregnancy.
- Normal hematologic changes of pregnancy include increased red blood cell (RBC) volume with physiologic thrombocytopenia and leukocytosis. Pregnancy is a state of hypercoagulability.
- Chronic hyperventilation and respiratory alkalosis occur during pregnancy.

- Elevated progesterone levels lead to smooth muscle relaxation and changes in the gastrointestinal tract.
- Human chorionic gonadotropin (hCG) structurally resembles thyroid-stimulating hormone (TSH), which can stimulate thyrotropin receptors and lead to physiologic TSH suppression and rise in thyroid hormones (T4 and T3). Maternal thyroid hormone is essential to fetal development in early gestation.
- Pregnancy is a state of physiologic hypercortisolism.
- Enlargement of the pituitary is primarily due to an increase in prolactin-producing lactotrophs.
- Insulin resistance increases throughout pregnancy.

PHYSIOLOGY OF PREGNANCY

Fluid balance

- During pregnancy, the maternal total volume increases due to the addition of the fetus, placenta, and amniotic fluid. Volume is also increased secondary to the intracellular fluid expansion of organs such as the uterus and breasts, increased maternal adipose tissue, and increased maternal blood volume to support a developing fetus.
- The body changes to a state of active water and sodium retention regulated by the posterior

pituitary and RAAS in order to support and accommodate these volume changes. This results in a chronic state of volume overload and contributes to maternal weight gain, hemodilution, physiologic anemia of pregnancy, and increased cardiac output. Overall blood volume increases by 1500–1600 mL during this time.[1,2]
- Water retention begins early in gestation through actions of anti-diuretic hormone (ADH), also known as arginine vasopressin (AVP), released by the posterior pituitary. The placenta releases gestational hormones including relaxin and nitrous oxide which

DOI: 10.1201/9781003027577-2

signal this increase in ADH secretion. After approximately 8 weeks gestation, ADH clearance also increases to balance volume levels to a relatively stable state. This becomes clinically significant if ADH clearance outweighs its secretion, leading to the potential unmasking of subclinical diabetes insipidus.[2]

- Sodium retention also occurs in early gestation. Approximately 900 mEq of sodium is accumulated throughout normal pregnancy. Most of this sodium is located in the amniotic fluid and will be lost at the time of delivery. Sodium levels increase due to the action of the RAAS, which is activated through cascades of hormones initiated by the posterior pituitary and placenta. The placenta releases nitrous oxide that decreases systemic vascular resistance (SVR), leading to a decrease in mean arterial pressure (MAP) and subsequent increases in renin, angiotensinogen, and angiotensin. These hormones increase by 4- to 5-fold and promote an increase in serum aldosterone levels at least 2-fold higher than the nonpregnant state in order to retain sodium and maintain intravascular volume.[1,3]

Cardiovascular

- The cardiovascular system undergoes significant changes during pregnancy which include effects on blood pressure, cardiac output, and cardiac structure. To accommodate the increased fluid volume, eccentric hypertrophy of the cardiac muscle occurs, which can take up to 6 months to return to normal.[1]
- Cardiac output is significantly altered in pregnancy, increasing by 30–50% compared to a nonpregnant state. This is due to a heart rate increase to an average of 90 beats per minute and a stroke volume increase to approximately 85 mL (from 65 mL). The steepest rise in cardiac output occurs early in pregnancy, then peaks and plateaus in the late second or early third trimester. This increase in cardiac output is needed to supply an increasing amount of blood flow to the uterus. During pregnancy, the uterus will receive 10–20% of the cardiac output versus 1–2% in the nonpregnant state. Other important organs also affected by the increased cardiac output include the kidneys, brain, skin, breasts, and coronary arteries.[4,5]

- Position changes in pregnancy affect cardiac output secondary to the gravid uterus compressing the inferior vena cava later in gestation. During labor, contractions increase the output by an additional 10% in early labor and up to 50% toward the end of the first stage of labor. An additional 10–20% increase occurs in the first 30 minutes after delivery.[5,6]
- Despite a large increase in cardiac output, the blood pressure (BP) early in pregnancy decreases secondary to decreased SVR by mechanisms discussed earlier. This change occurs until mid-pregnancy, after which the BP slowly rises.

Hematologic

- Blood volume increases in pregnancy from about 6 weeks until 30–34 weeks of gestation, after which it plateaus. The rise constitutes a 40–50% expansion in blood volume, secondary to increases in both plasma volume and RBC mass. As plasma volume can increase faster than RBC mass, this can lead to a physiologic anemia of pregnancy. The RBC mass is able to increase by 20% without oral iron supplementation and up to 30% with oral iron supplementation. Iron demands throughout the duration of pregnancy (assuming no iron deficiency prior to conception) are equivalent to approximately 1000 mg. Half of this (500 mg) is used to increase RBC mass, 300 mg is used by the developing fetus and placenta, and 200 mg assists in compensating for normal daily losses.[7]
- Changes in platelets and leukocytes also occur during pregnancy.
  - There is a decrease in platelet count secondary to a dilutional effect as well as increased destruction. Up to 8% of women will experience gestational thrombocytopenia. Platelets usually return to baseline approximately 1–2 weeks postpartum.
  - Pregnancy also induces a state of leukocytosis, with the white blood cell (WBC) count rising up to 20,000–30,000 during labor. The reason for this increase is unclear but thought to be secondary to increased estrogen and cortisol. Like platelets, the WBC count returns to normal 1–2 weeks postpartum.[8]

- Pregnancy is a state of hypercoagulability to defend against postpartum hemorrhage and the large amount of blood loss that occurs with delivery (500–1000 mL). Procoagulant factors increase, whereas natural inhibitors of coagulation and fibrinolysis decrease. While these mechanisms are important to avoid excessive blood loss during delivery, these changes can also increase the risk of venous thromboembolism up to 5- to 6-fold.

Respiratory

- Changes in chest wall dimensions during pregnancy can be attributed to both mechanical pressures from the enlarging uterus and from progesterone causing relaxation of ligaments within the chest wall. The diaphragm rises approximately 4 cm in pregnancy. Total lung capacity is decreased by 5%, while the functional residual capacity (FRC) is decreased by 20%. As a result of the FRC decrease, the inspiratory capacity and tidal volume (TV) increase by about 5–10%. The increase in TV with a relatively unchanged respiratory rate leads to a rise in minute ventilation up to 40%. This leads to a state of chronic hyperventilation and physiologic respiratory alkalosis.[9]

Renal and urinary

- Due to secondary effects of progesterone and ureteral compression, both renal length and diameter of the collecting system of the kidney increase. The bladder is also affected by uterine compression, leading to urinary frequency and urgency.
- Nitrous oxide and relaxin from the placenta are thought to alter renal physiology. These hormones decrease vascular resistance in the glomerular arteries, leading to increased GFR up to 50% and renal plasma flow (RPF) up to 75%. This raises serum creatinine clearance, resulting in a lower baseline creatinine in pregnancy. Likewise, blood urea nitrogen (BUN) and uric acid levels also decline.
- The increase in GFR alters the excretion of electrolytes and nutrients. Glucose, protein, albumin, amino acids, and calcium excretion are all increased. As a result of the respiratory alkalosis previously mentioned, the excretion of bicarbonate also increases. The rise in progesterone levels in pregnancy allows the kidneys to retain potassium, with excess potassium stored in the fetus and placenta.[1,10]

Gastrointestinal

- Progesterone leads to relaxation of smooth muscle, resulting in multiple physiologic changes in the GI system. Affected organs include the lower esophageal sphincter and stomach, leading to heartburn and nausea. Motility of the small intestine is also decreased, leading to constipation. Gallbladder emptying decreases, potentially increasing the risk of gallbladder sludge and gallstone formation.[1]

ENDOCRINE PHYSIOLOGY

Thyroid

- Despite many changes in thyroid hormones, pregnancy is a euthyroid state.
- Physiologic changes in thyroid hormone levels during pregnancy:
  - Thyroid-binding globulin (TBG) increases in the first trimester and plateaus later in the second trimester secondary to increased estrogen and hCG.
    - This raises total triiodothyronine (T3) and thyroxine (T4) levels.
    - Free T3 and free T4 remain relatively unchanged.
    - The small increase in total T4 concentration is known as gestational transient thyrotoxicosis and is necessary for adequate thyroid hormone to cross the placenta and aid in the development of the fetal neurologic system, as the fetus cannot produce its own thyroid hormone until approximately 12 weeks gestation.[1,11]
- Due to structural similarities between hCG and TSH, hCG can stimulate thyrotropin receptors on the thyroid gland in a manner similar to the action of TSH.
  - As hCG and increased estrogen levels stimulate a rise in T3 and T4, feedback leads to TSH suppression. TSH levels decrease by 18% in the first trimester,

5% in the second trimester, and 2% in the third trimester.

- Assuming adequate iodine intake, the thyroid minimally increases in size. As renal losses and fetal consumption lead to decreased iodine levels, it is recommended that maternal iodine intake increase from 100 mg/day to 250–290 mg/day to reduce the risk of maternal goiter.[1,11]

Adrenal

- Pregnancy is a state of physiologic hypercortisolism with changes including weight gain, striae, hyperglycemia, and fatigue.
- Increased steroid production is important for fetal growth and reproductive development.
- Increases in cortisol levels are caused by increased corticosteroid-releasing hormone (CRH). Outside of pregnancy, CRH is only produced by the hypothalamus. In pregnancy, it is also produced by the placenta and fetal membranes. Increased CRH signals the anterior pituitary to increase adrenocorticotropic hormone (ACTH), which in turn stimulates cortisol production from the adrenal glands. Increases in other adrenal hormones including aldosterone and deoxycorticosterone also occur.[1]

Pituitary

- The pituitary gland increases in size by approximately 36% during pregnancy, mainly due to increased lactotroph mass. The prolactin-producing lactotroph cells of the anterior pituitary cause a rise of prolactin up to 10 times the normal prepregnancy level by the end of the third trimester. In non-lactating women, the prolactin levels normalize by 3 months postpartum but may vary significantly among nursing mothers.
- Luteinizing hormone (LH) and follicle-stimulating hormone (FSH) are suppressed via negative feedback inhibition by elevated estrogen, progesterone, and inhibin levels.
- Growth hormone is suppressed due to negative feedback by placental growth hormone release.[12]
- Posterior pituitary release of ADH and oxytocin increases, with oxytocin peaking in the second trimester.[1]

Metabolic changes

- Significant changes in carbohydrate metabolism are required during pregnancy to support glucose demand in the developing fetus and placenta. Increased glucose requirements lead to increased insulin production. Hypertrophy and hyperplasia of the β-cells in the maternal pancreatic islets of Langerhans occur due to the increased demand for insulin. If insulin secretion cannot meet the increased glucose demands, gestational diabetes can develop.
- Lipid metabolism is also affected in pregnancy. There is a gradual increase in total triglycerides, total cholesterol, and low-density lipoprotein (LDL) concentration by mechanisms not well understood. No long-term risk factors have been identified from physiologic increases in lipids during pregnancy.[13]

REFERENCES

1. Gabbe, SG: Obstetrics: Normal and Problem Pregnancies. 7th ed. Philadelphia, PA: Elsevier, Inc; 2017; pp. 38–63.
2. Gunderson EP, Sternfeld B, Wellons MF, et al: Childbearing may increase visceral adipose tissue independent of overall increase in body fat. Obesity (Silver Spring) 2008; 16: pp. 1078–1084.
3. Duvekot JJ, Cheriex EC, Pieters FA, Menheere PP, Peeters LH: Early pregnancy changes in hemodynamics and volume homeostasis are consecutive adjustments triggered by a primary fall in systemic vascular tone. Am J Obstet Gynecol 1993; 169: pp. 1382–1392.
4. Sanghavi M, Rutherford JD: Cardiovascular physiology of pregnancy. Circulation 2014; 130: pp. 1003–1008.
5. Lee W, Rokey R, Miller J, Cotton DB: Maternal hemodynamic effects of uterine contractions by M-mode and pulsed-Doppler echocardiography. Am J Obstet Gynecol 1989; 161: pp. 974–977.
6. Robson SC, Hunter S, Boys RJ, Dunlop W: Serial study of factors influencing changes in cardiac output during human pregnancy. Am J Physiol 1989; 256: pp. H1060–H1065.
7. Pritchard J, Baldwin R, Dickey J: Blood volume changes in pregnancy and the

puerperium, II. Red blood cell loss and changes in apparent blood volume during and following vaginal delivery, cesarean section, and cesarean section plus total hysterectomy. Am J Obstet Gynecol 1962; 84: p. 1271.

8. Pitkin R, Witte D: Platelet and leukocyte counts in pregnancy. J Am Med Assoc 1979; 242: pp. 2696–2698.

9. Harirah HM, Donia SE, Nasrallah FK, Saade GR, Belfort MA: Effect of gestational age and position on peak expiratory flow rate: A longitudinal study. Obstet Gynecol 2005; 105: pp. 372–376.

10. Lindheimer M, Davison J, Katz A: The kidney and hypertension in pregnancy: Twenty exciting years. Semin Nephrol 2001; 21: pp. 173–189.

11. Glinoer D: The regulation of thyroid function in pregnancy: Pathways of endocrine adaptation from physiology. Endocr Rev 2014; 18: pp. 404–433.

12. Prager D, Braunstein GD: Pituitary disorders during pregnancy. Endocrinol Metab Clin North Am 1995; 24: pp. 1–14.

13. Phelps RL, Metzger BE, Freinkel N: Carbohydrate metabolism in pregnancy. XVII. Diurnal profiles of plasma glucose, insulin, free fatty acids, triglycerides, cholesterol, and individual amino acids in late normal pregnancy. Am J Obstet Gynecol 1981; 140: pp. 730–736.

Hormonal physiology of lactation

RAWAN EL-AMIN, LOREN CUSTER, AND JENNIFER SILK

KEY POINTS

- Lactogenesis involves the onset of milk production and secretion secondary to maturation of alveolar milk-producing cells.
- Prolactin produced by the anterior pituitary gland is the primary hormone for promoting milk production.

- Oxytocin produced in the hypothalamus and released by the posterior pituitary gland is responsible for milk letdown and secretion.

PHYSIOLOGY OF LACTATION

Anatomy and development of breasts

- Female breast development begins in utero during embryogenesis, matures during puberty, and differentiates during pregnancy and subsequent lactation. Mammary glands develop from the ectodermal ridge beginning as early as 7 weeks gestation.[1] During puberty, hypothalamic gonadotropin-releasing hormone (GnRH), follicle-stimulating hormone (FSH), and luteinizing hormone (LH) influence breast development.
- Breast tissue is comprised of epithelial and stromal components. The epithelial component contains branching ducts to connect the lobules to the nipple. Each mammary gland is composed of lobes containing lobules with numerous alveoli. The epithelium of the alveoli produces milk. The alveoli are surrounded by myoepithelial cells, which contract and allow milk flow along the ducts of the nipple. The stroma contains adipose and fibrous connective tissue.

- Sensory nerves to the nipple initiate the afferent neurologic pathway for milk ejection. There is no motor innervation to the myoepithelial cells or mammary epithelium; therefore, milk production and excretion are independent of neural stimulation.[1]
- Further duct development occurs under the influence of human chorionic gonadotropin (hCG) with expansion of lobules in the later stages of pregnancy. In preparation for milk production and secretion, the glandular epithelial component of breasts supersedes the stromal component. This is further regulated by estrogen, progesterone, prolactin, growth hormone, insulin, glucocorticoids, and local hormones within the breast tissue.[1] To support this change in breast composition and functionality, mammary blood flow doubles in pregnancy and continues postpartum during lactation.
- Mammary tissue can regress after pregnancy and re-differentiate in subsequent pregnancy as a response to hormonal changes.

DOI: 10.1201/9781003027577-3

Lactogenesis

- Lactogenesis involves the onset of milk production and secretion secondary to maturation of alveolar milk-producing cells.
  - The first stage begins with the morphologic differentiation of mammary epithelial cells during mid-pregnancy to support production of colostrum.[2] This stage is inhibited from further progression by high levels of progesterone during pregnancy.
  - The transition to stage two occurs at parturition when the placenta is delivered and levels of progesterone, estrogen, and human placental lactogen (hPL) decrease while prolactin levels remain high, possibly corresponding to increased cortisol and insulin levels. As the inhibitory influence of progesterone is no longer present, α-lactalbumin production increases. This stimulates the enzyme lactose synthase to increase lactose and milk production.[3] Thyroid hormones can also enhance the secretion of lactalbumin.
  - Stage two of lactogenesis can be altered in patients with diabetes, elevated cortisol induced by stress during late stages of labor, cesarean delivery, and retained products of conception including delayed placenta extraction.[1]
- During the first 2–4 days after delivery when progesterone levels decline, colostrum continues to be secreted. Within the first week postpartum, a change from endocrine to autocrine control of milk production and secretion occurs.
- Within the first 2 weeks after delivery, colostrum is followed by transitional milk secretion and finally by mature milk. This evolution of milk production and component concentrations is under the control of biosynthetic enzymes including fatty acid synthetase and acetyl-CoA carboxylase, as well as milk protein genes such as α-lactalbumin.[1] Galactopoiesis is maintained by this autocrine supply and demand process.

Milk production

- Milk synthesis and subsequent secretion fall into five generalized categories[4]:
  - Plasma components and leukocytes via the paracellular pathway
  - Exocytosis of lactose and milk protein
  - Apocrine secretion of milk fat globules
  - Pinocytosis-exocytosis of immunoglobulins
  - Secretion of water and ions across the apical membrane
- Milk components are absorbed in the maternal gastrointestinal tract or produced in the maternal liver with glucose being the main component. The volume and concentration of breast milk varies with each feed and a significant portion of milk is produced during nursing itself. For example, the lipid content of milk increases the longer a women nurses during a feeding session, therefore altering the caloric intake of milk.[2]
- The composition of milk changes in the first 3 days postpartum as the concentrations of sodium and chloride decline and lactose increases. This occurs secondary to the closure of tight junctions inhibiting the paracellular pathway.[4] Lactoferrin and secretory immunoglobulin A (sIgA) are initially secreted in high volumes but fall by day 2 postpartum.
- Due to low vitamin K and vitamin D in breast milk, infants are typically given intramuscular vitamin K at birth and supplemental vitamin D while breastfeeding.

Hormonal control of milk production

PROLACTIN

- Prolactin, a pleiotropic hormone produced by the lactotroph cells in the anterior pituitary gland, is the primary hormone for promoting milk production. Prolactin levels remain high throughout pregnancy which aids in the development of mammary glandular ductal tissue and expansion of epithelial cells for milk production. Milk production is inhibited, however, secondary to persistently elevated levels of progesterone and estrogen during pregnancy which block the effects of prolactin. The secretion of prolactin is also directly affected by dopamine, a hypothalamic inhibitory hormone. After parturition, prolactin binds to membrane receptors in mammary alveolar epithelial cells to promote milk production.[2]
- Following delivery, prolactin is secreted in a pulsatile manner correlating directly with nipple stimulation. Prolactin levels rise each

time a baby suckles stimulating the alveoli to produce milk.[5] Frequent stimulation of the breasts is essential early in milk production when lactation is being established. The serum concentration of prolactin does not directly correlate with the volume of milk produced. Of note, prolactin production increases at night; therefore, nipple stimulation and breastfeeding at night promote further milk supply.

- Levels of prolactin are usually around 200 ng/mL at delivery and fall to about 35 ng/mL by 6 months postpartum.[2] Serum levels rise within seconds of nipple stimulation and can suppress LH and ovarian function if women nurse at least 8 times per 24 hours for 10–20 minutes per feed.

OXYTOCIN

- Oxytocin, a nonapeptide hormone produced by the hypothalamus and released by the posterior pituitary gland, is responsible for milk letdown and secretion. Nipple stimulation and infant suckling stimulate an afferent neuronal pathway to trigger the paraventricular nuclei of the hypothalamus to produce oxytocin and subsequently trigger release by the posterior pituitary. Oxytocin binds G-protein-coupled receptors on myoepithelial cells in the alveoli to contract and express milk.
- Nursing cues, including triggering sights, sounds, and smells, can also stimulate the production of oxytocin.[2] Physical, emotional, and psychological stressors can inhibit oxytocin release and decrease milk secretion.[1]
- Oxytocin also stimulates uterine contractions postpartum to reduce bleeding. Women may experience cramping and abdominal pain secondary to oxytocin release with breastfeeding resulting in subsequent uterine contractions.[5]
- Increasing levels of oxytocin results in release of gastrointestinal hormones to facilitate gastrointestinal motility, which increases absorption of substrates necessary for lactogenesis.

Lactation and reproduction

- During pregnancy, placental steroids suppress the hypothalamic-pituitary-gonadal axis resulting in low levels of LH and FSH.
- Postpartum, in patients who are not breastfeeding, pulsatile secretion of GnRH can return to normal within 6 weeks resulting in ovarian follicular development.
- If a patient is breastfeeding, FSH secretion can return to normal by 4 weeks, but LH often remains suppressed.[4] Ovarian function usually remains suppressed during breastfeeding due to lack of pulsatile LH and GnRH secretion secondary to persistently elevated prolactin levels, continued suckling stimulation, and maternal nutrition.[1]

Cessation of milk production

- A decrease in frequency of breastfeeding and volume of milk production results in the resolution of lactation. A reduction in breastfeeding to fewer than six episodes in 24 hours or volumes less than 400 mL in 24 hours results in decreased prolactin levels.[2] Within 1–2 days of no milk secretion, intraductal pressures increase, and milk within the ducts release lactation inhibitory factor. Lactation inhibitory factor initiates apoptosis of secretory epithelial cells and decreases milk production from alveolar cells.[4]

REFERENCES

1. Truchet S, Honvo-Houeto E. Physiology of milk secretion. Best practice & research clinical endocrinology & metabolism. Best Pract Res Clin Endocrinol Metab. 2017 Aug;31(4):367–384.
2. Gabbe S, Niebyl J, Galan H, Jauniaux E, Landon M, Simpson J, Driscoll D. Lactation and breastfeeding. In: Newton ER, editor. Obstetrics: Normal and problem pregnancies. 6th ed. Philadelphia, PA: Elsevier/Saunders; 2012; pp. 535–61.
3. Cunninghan FG, Leveno KJ, Bloom SL, Dashe JS, Hoffman BL, Casey BM, Spong CY. Williams obstetrics. 25th ed. New York: McGraw-Hill Education; 2018; pp. 656–9.
4. Neville M. Physiology of lactation. *Clinics in Perinatology*. 1999;26(2):251–79.
5. World Health Organization. Infant and young child feeding: Model chapter for textbooks for medical students and allied health professionals. 2009. World Health Organization. https://apps.who.int/iris/handle/10665/44117

CHAPTER 2

Diabetes Mellitus

2a

Overview of diabetes mellitus in pregnancy

ROHMA SHAMSI, JESSICA PERINI, AND NADIA BARGHOUTHI

KEY POINTS

- Both gestational and pregestational diabetes (PGD) are increasing in prevalence.
- Diabetes in pregnancy significantly raises the risk for maternal and fetal complications.
- Counseling patients about the risks of diabetes and uncontrolled glucose levels is essential for improving pregnancy outcomes.
- Appropriate diet, monitoring blood glucose levels, and medical management can improve glucose control in pregnancy.

EPIDEMIOLOGY

- The prevalence of diabetes mellitus (DM) in women of reproductive age is increasing. Consequently, the number of women with preexisting diabetes who become pregnant is also rising.
- Over 10% of pregnancies worldwide are affected by diabetes.[1]
- PGD refers to a diagnosis of diabetes made prior to pregnancy. This term includes both type I and type II DM.
  - PGD complicates approximately 1–2% of all pregnancies.[2]
  - Approximately 10–20% of women have a diagnosis of diabetes prior to pregnancy.[2]
- The most common type of diabetes during pregnancy is gestational diabetes mellitus (GDM), accounting for up to 80–90% of all diabetes in pregnancy (see Chapter 2b).[1]
- The risk of congenital malformations increases with higher hemoglobin A1c (HbA1c) levels,

particularly in the first trimester. The best outcomes are typically associated with pre-pregnancy HbA1c values below 6–6.5%, while the risk of miscarriage or major malformations can be as high as 44% in those with an HbA1c of 12.8% or higher.[3]

PATHOPHYSIOLOGY

- Classification of diabetes
  - Most types of diabetes in pregnancy fit into one of the following classifications:
    - Type I DM is due to autoimmune destruction of the insulin-producing β-cells of the pancreas, leading to absolute insulin deficiency.
    - Type II DM is due to insufficient insulin production to maintain euglycemia in the setting of insulin resistance.
    - Gestational diabetes refers to any diabetes first diagnosed during pregnancy.

DOI: 10.1201/9781003027577-5

- Insulin resistance in pregnancy
  - First trimester:
    - In women with normal glucose metabolism, fasting glucose levels are lower than in the nonpregnant state due to increased uptake of glucose by the fetus and placenta. Postprandial sugars tend to be slightly higher than average due to the early effects of diabetogenic hormones produced by the placenta. In women with normal pancreatic function, insulin production is sufficient to meet the challenge of this physiologic insulin resistance created by these placental hormones and is sufficient to maintain normal glucose levels.
    - In women with preexisting diabetes, many may have no obvious changes in glucose levels during early pregnancy, but postprandial sugars may start to rise significantly.
  - Second and third trimesters:
    - Insulin resistance increases exponentially, plateauing toward the end of the third trimester.
    - Women with normal pancreatic function are generally able to produce enough insulin throughout pregnancy to compensate for the rise in insulin resistance and are able to maintain euglycemia.
    - Glucose levels, both fasting and postprandial, rise significantly in almost all women with diabetes.
  - Maternal and fetal effects of hyperglycemia and diabetes – please refer to Chapter 2c for detailed descriptions of adverse effects of diabetes during pregnancy.

DIAGNOSIS

- Diagnosis of diabetes prior to pregnancy is based on HbA1c ≥6.5%, fasting blood glucose ≥126 mg/dL, random glucose ≥200 mg/dL with symptoms of hyperglycemia, or any glucose ≥200 mg/dL after an oral glucose tolerance test.
- Diagnosis of diabetes during pregnancy is discussed in detail in Chapter 2b.

TREATMENT

- For women with preexisting diabetes planning pregnancy, optimizing glucose control prior to pregnancy provides the best chance of improved maternal and fetal outcomes.
- Prior to conception or as early during pregnancy as possible, women with preexisting diabetes should have the following:
  - Genetic screening offered.
  - Information provided regarding increased risk of maternal and fetal complications and screening options reviewed and offered.
  - Dilated eye exam to evaluate for retinopathy. The American Diabetes Association recommends dilated eye exams every trimester and over the first year postpartum, depending on the degree of any retinopathy.[4]
  - Appropriate vaccinations and nutritional counseling.
  - Assessment for and treatment of renal disease, neuropathy, and cardiovascular disease.
  - Thyroid-stimulating hormone (TSH) to evaluate thyroid function in women with type I DM.
- Regular visits with an obstetrician are essential throughout pregnancy to monitor maternal and fetal status as well as provide management of glycemic control.
- Diet, exercise, and medications can improve glucose control (see Chapter 2b).
- Women should perform self-monitoring of blood glucose (SMBG) 4–6 times per day.
- Oral medications, including glyburide and metformin, may be initiated if diet and exercise are not sufficient or if the patient cannot or will not use insulin.
- Insulins approved for use in pregnancy include detemir, neutral protamine Hagedorn (NPH), regular insulin (R), insulin aspart, and insulin lispro.
  - If a patient is using a different insulin prior to pregnancy and cannot or will not change to one of the above insulins, she may continue her previous insulin but must be informed that some insulin preparations are not FDA-approved for use during pregnancy so that an informed decision can be made. Small observational studies have not shown harm with the use of glargine insulin.[5]

- Glucose targets during pregnancy:
  - Fasting <95 mg/dL
  - 1-hour postprandial <140 mg/dL
  - 2-hour postprandial <120 mg/dL
  - HbA1c <6–6.5%
- Insulin requirements increase dramatically over the course of pregnancy but decline rapidly at parturition upon delivery of the placenta. Therefore, insulin doses may need to be reduced by up to 50% after delivery to prevent hypoglycemia.

REFERENCES

1. Stogianni A, et al. Obstetric and perinatal outcomes in pregnancies complicated by diabetes, and control pregnancies, in Kronoberg, Sweden. BMC Pregnancy Childbirth. 2019 May;19:159.
2. Hunt KJ, Schuller KL. The increasing prevalence of diabetes in pregnancy. Obstet Gynecol Clin North Am. 2007 Jun;34(2):173.
3. Greene MF, et al. First-trimester hemoglobin A1c and risk for major malformation and spontaneous abortion in diabetic pregnancy. Teratology. 1989 Mar;39(3):225–31.
4. Professional Practice Committee: Standards of Medical Care in Diabetes-2021. Diabetes Care. 2021 Jan;44(1):56.
5. Gallen IW, et al. Survey of glargine use in 115 pregnant women with type 1 diabetes. Diabet Med. 2008 Feb;25(2):165–9.

2b

Gestational diabetes

JEREMY SOULE

KEY POINTS

- Gestational diabetes mellitus (GDM) is common, occurring in approximately 10% of pregnancies.
- GDM increases the risk of maternal and fetal complications. Treatment reduces risk, mandating screening and therapy.
- Universal screening in the United States (US) is performed at gestational weeks 24–28; higher risk women are considered for earlier assessment of preexisting type II DM.

- Lifestyle measures including diet and exercise are foundational to the treatment of GDM.
- When needed, pharmacotherapy using insulin is generally preferred. Although controversial, metformin and glyburide are increasingly used.
- Postpartum women with GDM have an increased risk of developing type II DM. Lifelong surveillance with glucose monitoring is recommended.

EPIDEMIOLOGY

- GDM, defined as glucose intolerance developing or first recognized in pregnancy, is an important cause of pregnancy complications and increases the risk of preeclampsia, fetal macrosomia, shoulder dystocia, cesarean section, neonatal hypoglycemia, and other complications.[1,2]
- GDM is common, although the exact prevalence is clouded by imperfect data sources, differing diagnostic criteria, and changing prevalence over time and between populations. Worldwide, there is a marked variation in the prevalence of GDM, ranging from 1 to 45% of pregnancies.[3]
- Prevalence of GDM increased 56% between 2000 and 2010, according to CDC reporting of International Classification of Diseases, Ninth

Revision, Clinical Modification (ICD-9-CM) hospital admission data.[4]
- Prevalence in the United States was 4.6% by birth certificate data and 8.7% by Pregnancy Risk Assessment Monitoring System (PRAMS) questionnaires, with prevalence increasing with[5]:
  - Advancing age
  - Asian, Black, and Hispanic background
  - Increasing parity
  - Lower socioeconomic status
- Additional factors which increase the risk of GDM include[1,6]:
  - Obesity
  - Family history of diabetes
  - Past delivery of a macrosomic infant
  - History of dysglycemia without overt diabetes
  - Dyslipidemia

DOI: 10.1201/9781003027577-6

- Insulin resistance
- Physical inactivity
- Type II DM and GDM share risk factors, and GDM itself is highly predictive of later type II DM, as discussed below in postpartum follow-up.

PATHOPHYSIOLOGY

- Most cases of gestational diabetes develop in the setting of insulin resistance and risk factors shared with type II DM; however, autoimmune, monogenic (previously known as maturity-onset diabetes in youth, or MODY), and other less common forms of diabetes are infrequently first recognized in pregnancy.[7,8]
- Insulin resistance increases in the later weeks of normal pregnancy in step with increasing hormones from the placenta (lactogen and growth hormone) and mother (prolactin, progesterone, and cortisol), which in turn mildly increase maternal glycemia to putatively support fetal growth.[9–11]
- Women without GDM can overcome increasing insulin resistance and blunt hyperglycemia with increased insulin release. Compared to pregnancies uncomplicated by diabetes, women with GDM have increased insulin resistance and inability to control hyperglycemia despite increased insulin secretion.[11]
- Animal and genetic studies suggest mild deficits in the number and function of β-cells may be unmasked by the stress of pregnancy.[8] Thus, like type II DM, a combination of insulin resistance and a relative insulin deficiency participate in the pathogenesis of GDM.

DIAGNOSIS

Pregestational diabetes assessment

- Although GDM usually manifests early in the third trimester (screening is performed between 24 and 28 weeks gestation), the ongoing epidemic of type II DM has led to an increase in the number of women conceiving with preexisting but undiagnosed diabetes.
- As untreated hyperglycemia increases the risk for fetal malformations and other complications, testing for undiagnosed diabetes earlier

in pregnancy offers an opportunity to improve outcomes.

- The American Diabetes Association (ADA) and American College of Obstetrics and Gynecology (ACOG) recommend testing at the first prenatal visit for prediabetes and diabetes in patients with risk factors for type II DM.[1,12] Risk factors include the following:
  - GDM in prior pregnancy
  - Prediabetes as defined by[1]:
    - Impaired fasting glucose 100–125 mg/dL *or*
    - Impaired glucose tolerance with 2-hour postprandial glucose 140–199 mg/dL *or*
    - HbA1c 5.7–6.4%
  - BMI ≥25 kg/m² (≥23 kg/m² in Asian Americans)
  - First-degree family history of diabetes
  - Higher-risk ethnicity (African American, Hispanic, Asian, Pacific Islander)
  - History of vascular disease, hypertension, dyslipidemia, and polycystic ovarian syndrome
  - Physical inactivity
  - Evidence of insulin resistance such as acanthosis nigricans
  - Advancing age
- Although many obstetricians use standard screening procedures for GDM discussed below, diagnostic criteria for DM used outside of pregnancy may be used in earlier pregnancy[1,12]:
  - HbA1c ≥ 6.5% *or*
  - Fasting plasma glucose ≥126 mg/dL *or*
  - Random plasma glucose ≥200 mg/dL with symptoms of hyperglycemia *or*
  - 2-hour post 75-g oral glucose tolerance test (OGTT) glucose ≥200 mg/dL
- HbA1c is insufficiently sensitive to diagnose diabetes in pregnancy when used alone; fasting glucose measures and glucose tolerance testing should also be used.[12]

Screening for GDM

- The Hyperglycemia and Adverse Pregnancy Outcomes (HAPO) study assessed associations between maternal glycemia and complications in over 25,000 pregnancies with a one-step 75-g OGTT and showed increasing glycemia presents a continuum risk with no clear glucose threshold effect on complication risks.[13] Without a clear biological threshold between glycemia and risk, diagnostic criteria balance the burden of screening and treatment with improved pregnancy outcomes.

- In the United States, both two-step and one-step approaches are utilized (Tables 2b.1 and 2b.2).
  - Compared to the less stringent two-step approach, the one-step test identifies women with a lower but still elevated risk of pregnancy complications as well as postpartum maternal type II DM. ACOG argues the one-step approach increases diagnosis of GDM several-fold with unclear benefit, while the ADA notes that the vast majority of women with milder hyperglycemia are managed with lifestyle interventions only.

- The one-step approach is recommended by the International Association of Diabetes and Pregnancy Study Group (IADPSG), while the ADA deems either approach acceptable.[12,14]
- ACOG and the 2013 National Institute of Child Health and Human Development Consensus Development Conference on Diagnosing Gestational Diabetes support two-step testing, which avoids fasting in the screening phase (step 1); this approach is commonly used in clinical practice.[1,12,14]
- These criteria are based on outcomes in the HAPO trial, where glucose levels at these thresholds were associated with a 1.75 increased risk above mean in adverse outcomes (birth weight >90th percentile for gestational age, cesarean delivery, neonatal hypoglycemia, and cord-blood serum C-peptide level >90th percentile).[14]

Table 2b.1 Screening recommendations for GDM of different societies

Organization	Timing of screening	Method
American Diabetes Association (ADA)	24–28 weeks gestation	A. Two step: 50-g OGTT in a non-fasting state • If blood glucose at 1 hour >140 mg/dL, proceed to fasting OGTT with 100-g glucose load and blood glucose measurements at 1, 2, and 3 hours B. One step: 75-g OGTT with blood glucose measurements at 1 and 2 hours
Endocrine Society	First prenatal visit and 24–28 weeks gestation	• Universal screening at the first prenatal visit for all women who are not known to have diabetes using fasting plasma glucose levels, HbA1c, or random plasma glucose measurement • Testing for GDM at 24–28 weeks with 2-hour 75-g OGTT
USPSTF	24–28 weeks gestation	A. Two step (preferable): non-fasting 50-g OGTT • If the screening threshold is met (glucose level >130, 135, or 140 mg/dL, depending on lab assay), then proceed to 100-g OGTT with blood glucose measurements at 1, 2, and 3 hours B. One step: 75-g OGTT with blood glucose measurements at 1 and 2 hours

Table 2b.2 Normal plasma glucose levels following glucose load

Time	Carpenter/ Coustan glucose (mg/dL)	National Diabetes Data Group glucose (mg/dL)
Fasting	<95	<105
1 hour	<180	<190
2 hours	<155	<165
3 hours	<140	<145

Other diagnostic tests for GDM

- In women with hyperemesis, history of gastric bypass surgery, or those unable to tolerate glucose tolerance testing, checking HbA1c and assessing fasting and 1-hour postprandial glucose every several weeks in later pregnancy can be used to assess for dysglycemia.[15]

TREATMENT

Rationale for therapy

- Although GDM complications were long recognized, clinical trial data supporting treatment of GDM were not available until the 2005 publication of the Australian Carbohydrate Intolerance Study in Pregnant Women (ACHOIS) and the 2009 publication of the US-based study by Landon et al.[16,17] Both studies included women with milder GDM, with intervention groups receiving dietary therapy, glucose self-monitoring, and insulin when lifestyle measures failed.
- Treatment of glucose to stringent targets decreased serious perinatal complications such as shoulder dystocia and nerve palsies, macrosomia, and maternal hypertension. The ACHOIS study also showed treatment lessened depression symptoms and improved health-related quality of life, allaying concerns that aggressive screening and treatment for milder GDM might have adverse psychological impacts.

Goals of therapy

- ACOG and ADA recommended self-monitored glucose targets from the Fifth International Workshop–Conference on GDM[14]

- Fasting glucose <95 mg/dL *and*
- One-hour postprandial glucose <140 mg/dL *or* 2-hour postprandial glucose <120 mg/dL
- Self-monitored blood glucose (SMBG) testing
  - Should be performed at least 4 times daily, including fasting and postprandially
  - Testing frequency can be decreased if glucose levels are within target but should continue at varying times of each day with sufficient data to profile glycemia throughout the day[1]
- HbA1c
  - Should serve as a complementary target only, with use secondary to SMBG
  - Does not capture postprandial hyperglycemia or episodes of hypoglycemia
  - Prone to variability
  - Individualized targets:
    - 6–7% is reasonable in early pregnancy.
    - <6% can be considered if achievable without undue hypoglycemia.[12]
- Continuous glucose monitoring (CGM)
  - ADA supports a role for CGM to complement SMBG in pregnancy.
  - Some CGM trials in pregnant women with diabetes have demonstrated the following:
    - Reductions in HbA1c without increased hypoglycemia.
    - Reductions in adverse perinatal outcomes.
    - Limitations: Much of the data derives from women with pregestational diabetes rather than GDM.[18–21]

Lifestyle interventions

- Lifestyle measures are central to the treatment of GDM and are sufficient to control glucose levels in a large majority of patients. Nutrition therapy, without the protocol-driven need for the addition of insulin, was used in 80% of women in the ACHOIS study and 92% of women in the US-based study by Landon.[16,17]

Diet

- Medical nutritional therapy is recognized as fundamental to GDM care; however, there are little data to guide specific interventions.[22]

- ADA and Endocrine Society (ES) support gestational weight gain targets of the 2009 Institute of Medicine recommendations[23]:
  - Weight gain targets of 0.5–2 kg in the first trimester, based on prepregnancy BMI
  - Underweight (BMI <18.5) prior to pregnancy: 0.44–0.58 kg/week in last two trimesters
  - Normal weight (BMI 18.5–24.9) prior to pregnancy: 0.35–0.5 kg/week
  - Overweight (BMI 25–29.9) prior to pregnancy: 0.23–0.33 kg/week
  - Obese (BMI ≥30) prior to pregnancy: 0.17–0.27 kg/week
- Where available, women ideally receive guidance from a registered dietician.[12]
- Caloric intake should be reduced in overweight and obese women but sufficient to avoid ketosis and support fetal and maternal health, with a suggested minimum daily caloric intake of 1600–1800 calories.[24]
- In regard to nutritional content, although there is little data to guide specific recommendations, some studies suggest decreased risk of macrosomia with low glycemic index diets.[25]
- ES recommends curtailing carbohydrate intake to 35–40% of total calories, while ACOG and ADA make no formal recommendation on total carbohydrate restriction.
  - ADA recommends at least 175 g of carbohydrate, 71 g of protein, and 28 g of fiber daily, while noting simple carbohydrates increase postprandial glucose.
  - ACOG recommends distributing carbohydrates between 3 meals and 2–3 snacks in order to limit postprandial glucose excursions that can occur with larger carbohydrate loads.

Exercise

- Although a recent Cochrane study found exercise reduced glucose levels in GDM, there were insufficient data to assess perinatal outcomes.[26]
- ADA, ACOG, and ES all recommend regular moderate exercise, e.g., 30 minutes of daily exercise at least 5 days per week.

Pharmacotherapy

- Pharmacotherapy is initiated for women not meeting goals of therapy with lifestyle measures.

- Insulin does not cross the placenta, is the most studied pharmacologic class in pregnancy, and is preferred over other therapies, including metformin and sulfonylureas.
- Metformin and glyburide can be used in some situations, such as refusal or inability to adhere to insulin therapy. The Society for Maternal-Fetal Medicine, in a rebuttal to ACOG guideline preference for insulin, recognizes metformin as an acceptable first-line pharmacologic alternative to insulin, citing efficacy, patient preference, and outcomes as discussed below.[27]
- Insulin
  - Generally, both long-acting and rapid-acting insulins are used to provide fasting (basal) and postprandial glucose control, respectively.
  - Citing a lack of quality data, a Cochrane review could not recommend any specific insulin type or regimen.[28]
  - Insulin safety data in pregnancy:
    - Lispro, aspart, and detemir have reassuring animal studies and trials in human pregnancy and, along with conventional human regular and Neutral Protamine Hagedorn (NPH) insulins, were classified as pregnancy category B prior to the 2015 revision of FDA pregnancy categories.[29]
    - Less studied in human pregnancy, inhaled insulin, glulisine, degludec, and glargine U-100 were previously category C.
    - For the more recently released (post-2015) insulins, glargine U-300 and the Fiasp® formulation of aspart, labeling notes a lack of clear data to inform maternal and fetal risk while also citing specific animal and human data.
    - Label updates for insulins with pre-2015 FDA categorizations have adopted similar insulin-specific labeling. Compared to regular insulin, which is optimally delivered at least 10–15 minutes before meals, lispro and aspart are preferred by ACOG for offering better postprandial control when given immediately before a meal.[1]
  - Regarding dose and regimen, specific society level guidelines are lacking, but

the California Diabetes and Pregnancy Program (CDAPP): Sweet Success is often quoted.[15,30]

- For more severe hyperglycemia, CDAPP recommends 0.6–1.0 units of insulin per kg/day divided as 50% for meals with a rapid-acting insulin and 50% for basal needs with an intermediate insulin (NPH) given twice daily or a once daily long-acting insulin.
- For milder fasting hyperglycemia, such as fasting glucose elevations to <120 mg/dL, bedtime NPH doses of 8–20 units can be initiated.
- For milder postprandial excursions (<180 mg/dL), 2–4 units of rapid-acting insulin can be used premeal.

- Regardless of regimen, patients starting insulin should be educated about managing hypoglycemia and initially seen frequently, usually at least weekly, for SMBG-based adjustments of insulin and dietary regimens.
- During labor, the goal is to normalize glucose to 70–110 mg/dL, as this will reduce the risk of neonatal hypoglycemia.[15]
- Many women with GDM, especially those treated with diet and not requiring pharmacotherapy, can be managed through labor without medication.
- When hyperglycemia develops (glucose >100 mg/dL), management includes intravenous insulin and fluid algorithms (see CDAPP reference).[15]
- After delivery, many women with GDM will not need insulin. However, glucose levels should be monitored and non-insulin therapies considered if hyperglycemia persists.

- Glyburide
  - The sulfonylurea glyburide has been studied in pregnancy and offers the convenience of an inexpensive oral therapy.
  - Despite guideline preference for insulin from ACOG and ADA, glyburide use has increased. According to studies of registry data, glyburide use in pregnancy surpasses insulin in the United States.[31]
  - Glyburide crosses the placenta.
  - Long-term outcome data in offspring of women who used glyburide through pregnancy is lacking.

- Meta-analysis data of glyburide versus insulin raised concerns of fetal and maternal hypoglycemia and fetal macrosomia. In addition, a recent, larger non-inferiority clinical trial demonstrated that glyburide failed to show equivalence to insulin in perinatal outcomes.[1,32]
- Glyburide in GDM is initiated at low doses, 1.25–2.5 mg daily, and titrated for effect to a maximum dose of 10 mg twice daily.
- Hypoglycemia is reduced by dosing glyburide 1 hour prior to meals.[15]
- Patients treated with glyburide should be educated on hypoglycemia recognition and management.
- Treatment failure with the need for progression to insulin therapy occurred in 6–18% of women in various trials.[33]

- Metformin
  - Like glyburide, metformin is an inexpensive oral medication and is increasingly used in pregnancy despite ADA and ACOG preference for insulin therapy.[31]
  - Even with its gastrointestinal side effects, study data suggest women prefer metformin to insulin therapy.[33]
  - Although meta-analysis has been largely reassuring regarding metformin versus insulin use in GDM, with less maternal weight gain and the trend toward less neonatal hyperglycemia, some studies show metformin results in more preterm delivery and offspring with increased childhood weight gain.[12,34]
  - Metformin crosses the placenta.
  - ADA recommends against metformin in pregnancies complicated by hypertension, preeclampsia, or otherwise at risk for intrauterine growth restriction (IUGR).[12]
  - ADA also cites a risk for acidosis and IUGR in the setting of placental insufficiency with metformin use.[12]
  - Metformin in GDM is initiated at 500 mg once or twice daily with food and adjusted based on tolerance to a maximal daily dose of 2500 mg.
  - Metformin should not be used in renal insufficiency and should be held in the event of major illness or surgery.
  - Glucose should be closely monitored as failure of metformin is common, with the

need for insulin rescue seen in up to 46% of women.[35]

Postpartum management

- GDM greatly increases the risk of later development of type II DM by approximately 7-fold.[36] This risk mandates ongoing assessment for type II DM after GDM.
  - ADA and ACOG both recommend testing at 4–12 weeks postpartum with a fasting glucose and a 75-g OGTT in preference to HbA1c or fasting glucose alone.[1,12] Positive results mandate treatment for diabetes.
  - Women with impaired fasting glucose or impaired glucose tolerance have prediabetes and should be counseled regarding diet, exercise, and weight loss.[12] Metformin can also be considered as first-line therapy.[37]
  - Women with normal testing at 4–12 weeks postpartum still require indefinite follow-up, with ADA suggesting testing every 1–3 years using any ADA recommended glycemic test.[12]
- For subsequent pregnancies, women with a history of GDM should be instructed to seek preconception counseling and assessment of glycemia.[1,12]

REFERENCES

1. Caughey AB, Turrentine M. Committee on Practice Bulletins—Obstetrics. ACOG Practice Bulletin No. 190: Gestational Diabetes Mellitus. *Obstet Gynecol*. 2018 Feb;131(2):e49–e64.
2. Mack LR, Tomich PG. Gestational diabetes: Diagnosis, classification, and clinical care. *Obstet Gynecol Clin North Am*. 2017 Jun;44(2):207–217.
3. Agarwal MM, Dhatt GS, Othman Y. Gestational diabetes: Differences between the current international diagnostic criteria and implications of switching to IADPSG. *J Diabetes Complications*. 2015;29(4):544–549.
4. Buchanan TA, Xiang AH. Gestational diabetes mellitus. *J Clin Invest*. 2005;115(3):485–491.
5. DeSisto CL, Kim SY, Sharma AJ. Prevalence estimates of gestational diabetes mellitus in the United States, Pregnancy Risk Assessment Monitoring System (PRAMS), 2007–2010. *Prev Chronic Dis*. 2014;11:130415.
6. Zhang C, Rawal S, Chong YS. Risk factors for gestational diabetes: Is prevention possible? *Diabetologia*. 2016;59:1385–1390.
7. Bardenheier BH, Imperatore G, Gilboa SM, Geiss LS, Saydah SH, Devlin HM, Kim SY, Gregg EW. Trends in gestational diabetes among hospital deliveries in 19 U.S. States, 2000–2010. *Am J Prev Med*. 2015 Jul;49(1):12–19.
8. Plows JF, Stanley JL, Baker PN, Reynolds CM, Vickers MH. The pathophysiology of gestational diabetes mellitus. *Int J Mol Sci*. 2018 Oct;19(11):3342.
9. Ryan EA, Enns L. Role of gestational hormones in the induction of insulin resistance. *J Clin Endocrinol Metab*. 1988 Aug;67(2): 341–347.
10. Velegrakis A, Sfakiotaki M, Sifakis S. Human placental growth hormone in normal and abnormal fetal growth (Review). *J Matern Fetal Neonatal Med*. 2007 Sep;20(9): 651–659.
11. Catalano PM, Tyzbir ED, Roman NM, Amini SB, Sims EA. Longitudinal changes in insulin release and insulin resistance in nonobese pregnant women. *Am J Obstet Gynecol*. 1991 Dec;165(6 Pt 1):1667–1672.
12. American Diabetes Association. Classification and diagnosis of diabetes: Standards of medical care in diabetes—2020. *Diabetes Care*. 2020 Jan;43(Supplement 1):S14–S31.
13. HAPO Study Cooperative Research Group, Metzger BE, Lowe LP, Dyer AR, Trimble ER, Chaovarindr U, Coustan DR, Hadden DR, McCance DR, Hod M, McIntyre HD, Oats JJ, Persson B, Rogers MS, Sacks DA. Hyperglycemia and adverse pregnancy outcomes. *N Engl J Med*. 2008 May;358(19):1991–2002.
14. International Association of Diabetes and Pregnancy Study Groups Consensus Panel, Metzger BE, Gabbe SG, Persson B, Buchanan TA, Catalano PA, Damm P, Dyer AR, de Leiva A, Hod M, Kitzmiler JL, Lowe LP, McIntyre HD, Oats JJN, Omori Y, Schmidt MI. International Association of Diabetes and Pregnancy Study Groups recommendations on the

diagnosis and classification of hypergly-cemia in pregnancy. *Diabetes Care*. 2010 Mar;33(3):676–682.

15. Shields, L, Tsay, GS. Editors, California Diabetes and Pregnancy Program (CDAPP) Sweet Success Guidelines for Care. Developed with California Department of Public Health; Maternal, Child and Adolescent Health Division; revised edition, 2012 Jul:1–18.

16. Crowther CA, Hiller JE, Moss JR, McPhee AJ, Jeffries WS, Robinson JS. Australian Carbohydrate Intolerance Study in Pregnant Women (ACHOIS) Trial Group. Effect of treatment of gestational diabetes mellitus on pregnancy outcomes. *N Engl J Med*. 2005;352:2477–2486.

17. Landon MB, Spong CY, Thom E, Carpenter MW, Ramin SM, Casey B, Wapner RJ, Varner MW, Rouse DJ, Thorp JM Jr, Sciscione A, Catalano P, Harper M, Saade G, Lain KY, Sorokin Y, Peaceman AM, Tolosa JE, Anderson GB, Eunice Kennedy Shriver National Institute of Child Health and Human Development Maternal-Fetal Medicine Units Network. A multicenter, randomized trial of treatment for mild gestational diabetes. *N Engl J Med*. 2009 Oct;361(14):1339–1348.

18. Paramasivam SS, Chinna K, Singh AKK, Ratnasingam J, Ibrahim L, Lim LL, Tan ATB, Chan SP, Tan PC, Omar SZ, Bilous RW, Vethakkan SR. Continuous glucose moni-toring results in lower HbA1c in Malaysian women with insulin-treated gestational dia-betes: A randomized controlled trial. *Diabet Med*. 2018 Aug;35(8):1118–1129.

19. Voormolen DN, DeVries JH, Sanson RME, Heringa MP, de Valk HW, Kok M, van Loon AJ, Hoogenberg K, Bekedam DJ, Brouwer TCB, Porath M, Erdtsieck RJ, NijBijvank B, Kip H, van der Heijden OWH, Elving LD, Hermsen BB, Potter van Loon BJ, Rijnders RJP, Jansen HJ, Langenveld J, Akerboom BMC, Kiewiet RM, Naaktgeboren CA, Mol BWJ, Franx A, Evers IM. Continuous glucose monitoring during diabetic preg-nancy (GlucoMOMS): A multicentre ran-domized controlled trial. *Diabetes Obes Metab*. 2018 Aug;20(8):1894–1902. Epub 2018 May 8.

20. Feig DS, Donovan LE, Corcoy R, Murphy KE, Amiel SA, Hunt KF, Asztalos E, Barrett JFR, Sanchez JJ, de Leiva A, Hod M, Jovanovic L, Keely E, McManus R, Hutton EK, Meek CL, Stewart ZA, Wysocki T, O'Brien R, Ruedy K, Kollman C, Tomlinson G, Murphy HR, CONCEPTT Collaborative Group. Continuous glucose monitoring in pregnant women with type 1 diabetes (CONCEPTT): A multicentre international randomised controlled trial. *Lancet*. 2017 Nov;390(10110):2347–2359. doi: 10.1016/S0140-6736(17)32400-5. Epub 2017 Sep 15.

21. Murphy HR, Rayman G, Lewis K, Kelly S, Johal B, Duffield K, Fowler D, Campbell PJ, Temple RC. Effectiveness of continuous glucose monitoring in pregnant women with diabetes: Randomised clinical trial. *BMJ*. 2008 Sep;337:a1680.

22. Han S, Crowther CA, Middleton P, Heatley E. Different types of dietary advice for women with gestational diabetes mel-litus. *Cochrane Database Syst Rev*. 2013 Mar;28(3):CD009275.

23. Institute of Medicine and National Research Council. Weight Gain during Pregnancy: Reexamining the Guidelines. Washington, DC, National Academies Press, 2009.

24. Blumer I, Hadar E, Hadden DR, Jovanovič L, Mestman JH, Murad MH, and Yogev Y. Diabetes and pregnancy: An endocrine society clinical practice guideline. *J Clin Endocrinol Metab*. 2013;98:4227–4249.

25. Han S, Middleton P, Shepherd E, Van Ryswyk E, Crowther CA. Different types of dietary advice for women with gestational diabetes mellitus. *Cochrane Database Syst Rev*. 2017 Feb;2:CD009275.

26. Brown J, Ceysens G, Boulvain M. Exercise for pregnant women with gestational diabetes for improving maternal and fetal outcomes. *Cochrane Database Syst Rev*. 2017 Jun 22;6:CD012202.

27. Society of Maternal-Fetal Medicine (SMFM) Publications Committee. SMFM Statement: Pharmacological treatment of gestational diabetes. *Am J Obstet Gynecol*. 2018;218(5):B2–B4.

28. O'Neill SM, Kenny LC, Khashan AS, West HM, Smyth RM, Kearney PM. Different insu-lin types and regimens for pregnant women

with pre-existing diabetes. *Cochrane Database Syst Rev.* 2017 Feb 3;2:CD011880.

29. Blum AK. Insulin use in pregnancy: An update. *Diabetes Spectrum.* 2016 May;29(2):92–97.

30. Hone J, Jovanovič L. Approach to the patient with diabetes during pregnancy. *J Clin Endocrinol Metab.* 2010 Aug;95(8):3578–3585.

31. Cesta CE, Cohen JM, Pazzagli L, Bateman BT, Bröms G, Einarsdóttir K, Furu K, Havard A, Heino A, Hernandez-Diaz S, Huybrechts KF, Karlstad Ø, Kieler H, Li J, Leinonen MK, Gulseth HL, Tran D, Yu Y, Zoega H, Odsbu I1. Antidiabetic medication use during pregnancy: An international utilization study. *BMJ Open Diabetes Res Care.* 2019 Nov;7(1):e000759.

32. Sénat MV, Affres H, Letourneau A, Coustols-Valat M, Cazaubiel M, Legardeur H, Jacquier JF, Bourcigaux N, Simon E, Rod A, Héron I, Castera V, Sentilhes L, Bretelle F, Rolland C, Morin M, Deruelle P, De Carne C, Maillot F, Beucher G, Verspyck E, Desbriere R, Laboureau S, Mitanchez D, Bouyer J, Groupe de Recherche en Obstétrique et Gynécologie (GROG). Effect of glyburide vs subcutaneous insulin on perinatal complications among women with gestational diabetes: A randomized clinical trial. *JAMA.* 2018 May;319(17):1773–1780.

33. Balsells M, García-Patterson A, Solà I, Roqué M, Gich I, Corcoy R. Glibenclamide, metformin, and insulin for the treatment of gestational diabetes: A systematic review and meta-analysis. *BMJ.* 2015;350:h102.

34. Jiang YF, Chen XY, Ding T, Wang XF, Zhu ZN, Su SW. Comparative efficacy and safety of OADs in management of GDM: Network meta-analysis of randomized controlled trials. *J Clin Endocrinol Metab.* 2015 May;100(5):2071–2080.

35. Rowan JA, Hague WM, Gao W, Battin MR, Moore MP, MiG Trial Investigators. Metformin versus insulin for the treatment of gestational diabetes. *N Engl J Med.* 2008 May;358(19):2003–2015.

36. Bellamy L, Casas JP, Hingorani AD, Williams D. Type 2 diabetes mellitus after gestational diabetes: A systematic review and meta-analysis. *Lancet.* 2009 May;373(9677):1773–1779.

37. Ratner RE, Christophi CA, Metzger BE, Dabelea D, Bennett PH, Pi-Sunyer X, Fowler S, Kahn SE, The Diabetes Prevention Program Research Group. Prevention of diabetes in women with a history of gestational diabetes: Effects of metformin and lifestyle interventions. *J Clin Endocrinol Metab.* 2008 Dec;93(12):4774–4779.

Diabetic maternal and fetal complications

RASHI SANDOOJA AND JASMIN LEBASTCHI

KEY POINTS

- Gestational diabetes mellitus (GDM) is associated with multiple maternal and fetal complications.
- Women with GDM have an increased risk of developing diabetes later in life.
- Some studies suggest a correlation between maternal hyperglycemia and the development of gestational hypertension and preeclampsia.

- Fetal complications of diabetes in pregnancy include macrosomia, congenital malformations, and stillbirth.
- Long-term complications in children born to women with diabetes include obesity and possible later development of diabetes and cardiovascular disease.

MATERNAL COMPLICATIONS

- Gestational hypertension and preeclampsia:
  - Multiple mechanisms can contribute to the development of gestational hypertension.
    - Increased insulin resistance activates the sympathetic nervous system and increases endothelin receptors, leading to hypertension.
    - Hypertriglyceridemia associated with insulin resistance leads to endothelial dysfunction, reduced prostacyclin production, and interferes with nitric oxide-mediated vasodilation, further contributing to the development of hypertension.[1]
  - Pathophysiologic factors involved in pre-eclampsia can be linked to those of GDM.[2]

- Incidence of preeclampsia is up to 9.9% in diabetic pregnancies as compared to 4.3% in nondiabetic controls.[3]
    - Incidence of preeclampsia rises with the increasing severity of diabetes.
      - One study showed that the rate of preeclampsia increased from 7.8% in patients with mild hypergly-cemia (fasting blood sugar [FBS] <105 mg/dL) to 13.8% in those with severe hyperglycemia (FBS >105 mg/dL).[1]
    - Optimal glycemic control during pregnancy may reduce the rate of preeclampsia.
  - Patients with GDM who developed pre-eclampsia were significantly younger, with a higher nulliparity rate, and with higher rates of obesity.

DOI: 10.1201/9781003027577-7

- Perinatal mortality rates are approximately 60 per 1000 births among diabetic women with preeclampsia versus 3.3 per 1000 births for normotensive diabetic patients.[3]
- Other studies showed an indeterminate association between GDM and preeclampsia.[1,4]
- Higher rates of induction of labor and cesarean delivery are noted in women with GDM and preeclampsia.[5]
- Uncontrolled blood glucose levels secondary to GDM lead to future increased risk of:
  - Lipid disturbances
  - Elevated mean systolic blood pressure
  - Atherosclerotic disease including myocardial infarction[6,7]
  - Recurrence of GDM in subsequent pregnancies
  - Development of type II DM
    - Women with GDM have a 7-fold increased risk of developing type II DM in comparison to women with normoglycemic pregnancy.[6]
    - Cumulative incidence of type II DM increases markedly in the first 5 years after delivery, may reach up to 70% long term, but typically plateaus after 10 years postpartum.[8]
    - ADA recommends postpartum blood glucose testing at 6–8 weeks and every 3 years thereafter. Unfortunately, most who develop GDM are lost to follow-up and not screened after delivery.[9]
    - Genetic studies suggest that GDM and type II DM are similar in that the frequency of some alleles associated with type II DM is also increased in GDM.[10]
    - Potential risk factors for progression to type II DM include the following:
      - Obesity prior to and during pregnancy
      - Family history of diabetes
        - 34.6% of those who develop type II DM after GDM have a first degree relative with diabetes
      - Ethnicity
        - Asian and African Americans are at higher risk
      - Poor GDM glucose control

FETAL COMPLICATIONS

- Uncontrolled maternal hyperglycemia leads to increased transfer of maternal glucose through the placenta. However, maternal or exogenously administered insulin is unable to cross the placenta, leading to increased autonomous secretion of insulin by the fetal pancreas, increased utilization of glucose, and increased fetal adipose tissue leading to macrosomia. This is the basis of a majority of fetal complications due to maternal hyperglycemia.[11]
- Short-term complications
  - Macrosomia
    - Defined by excess body fat, increase in muscle mass, and organomegaly without increase in brain size.
    - Prevalence in developed countries is 5–20% with a recent increase to 15–25%.[12]
    - Increased glucose levels during OGTT are associated with birth weight >90th percentile.[13]
    - Genes for lipid transport and inflammatory pathways are upregulated in the placenta of women with GDM, increasing delivery of lipid substrates for fetal use, contributing to macrosomia and increased birth weight.[14]
    - Treatment of GDM with lifestyle modifications or insulin reduces rates of macrosomia.[15]
  - Congenital malformations and diabetic embryopathy:
    - Maternal hyperglycemia has teratogenic effects by the following mechanisms[16,17]:
      - Alterations in cell lipid metabolism, especially prostaglandin dysregulation, which affect membranogenesis and function
      - Excessive generation of reactive oxygen species due to mitochondrial dysfunction
      - Activation of programmed cell death or apoptosis
    - Patients with type I or II DM prior to pregnancy are significantly more likely to have a child with one or more birth defects as compared to pregnant

women who never had diabetes or developed diabetes late in pregnancy.[18]

- Infants born to those with pregestational diabetes are more likely to develop cardiac defects (transposition of great arteries, ventricular or atrial septal defects, coarctation of aorta, caudal regression syndrome), central nervous system anomalies (neural tube defect, anencephaly), gastrointestinal defects (duodenal and anal atresia, hypoplastic left colon), and genitourinary malformations.[18]
- Stringent glucose control prior to or early in pregnancy can significantly reduce the incidence of birth defects.[17]
- Perinatal death
  - All forms of diabetes during pregnancy are associated with an increased risk of stillbirth due to hypoxia and acidosis associated with anaerobic metabolism.[19]
- Neonatal respiratory distress syndrome
  - Maternal diabetes can increase the risk of meconium aspiration and transient tachypnea of the newborn, especially in babies born by cesarean delivery.
- Metabolic derangements
  - Neonatal hypoglycemia
    - Infants with excessive size at birth are more likely to develop hyperinsulinemia and hypoglycemia.[13]
    - Large for gestational age infants born to diabetic mothers should have frequent blood glucose checks on the first day after birth. Earlier and frequent breastfeeding is an effective strategy to prevent hypoglycemia in these babies.[16]
  - Neonatal hypocalcemia can be reduced with strict maternal diabetes management.[20]
  - Neonatal polycythemia and hyperbilirubinemia are associated with increased maternal glucose levels and increased fetal metabolic rate and glucose uptake, leading to an increase in tissue oxygen consumption and hypoxia. This is a potent stimulator of fetal erythropoietin, leading to

polycythemia, increased blood viscosity, and hyperbilirubinemia.
  - Often presents as lethargy, hypotonia, and irritability in the neonate
  - In severe cases, may present as seizures secondary to cerebral infarcts[16]

- Long-term complications
  - Obesity
    - The mechanisms by which in utero exposure to diabetes increases the risk of diabetes and obesity in offspring is not clearly understood. It may be attributed to increased fetal mass or alterations in fetal hormones secondary to hyperglycemia. Increased concentrations of insulin or fetal leptin levels seen in these offspring may also play a role.[21]
    - Children of Pima Indian women with GDM or preexisting type II DM were larger for gestational age at birth and heavier at every age, adjusted for height, as compared to those of nondiabetic women.[22,23]
    - In sibling studies among Pima Indians, those born to women with maternal diabetes had significantly higher body mass index (BMI) than their siblings who had not been exposed to diabetes in utero.[24]
    - In the United States, children born to women with GDM have a 17.1% increased risk of becoming overweight. Of children of women with GDM, 9.7% are overweight. This is in contrast to 6.6% of children whose mothers did not have diabetes.[25]
    - Obesity appears to be linked more to maternal glucose status than to maternal pregnancy weight. Neonates born to diabetic mothers with normal birth weight had a higher incidence of childhood obesity.[26]
  - Cardiovascular
    - Some studies suggest an increased risk of cardiovascular dysfunction later in life in offspring exposed to maternal DM.[16,27]

REFERENCES

1. Yogev Y, Xenakis EM, Langer O. The association between preeclampsia and the severity of gestational diabetes: the impact of glycemic control. *Am J Obstet Gynecol.* 2004;191(5):1655–1660.

2. Henry, OA, Beischer NA. 11 long-term implications of gestational diabetes for the mother. *Baillieres Clin Obstet Gynaecol.* 1991;5(2):461–483.

3. Garner PR, D'Alton ME, Dudley DK, Huard P, Hardie M. Preeclampsia in diabetic pregnancies. *Am J Obstet Gynecol.* 1990;163(2):505–508.

4. Schaffir JA, Lockwood CJ, Lapinski R, Yoon L, Alvarez M. Incidence of pregnancy-induced hypertension among gestational diabetics. *Am J Perinatol.* 1995;12(4):252–254.

5. Weissgerber TL, Mudd LM. Preeclampsia and diabetes. *Curr Diab Rep.* 2015;15(3):9.

6. Bellamy L, Casas JP, Hingorani AD, Williams D. Type 2 diabetes mellitus after gestational diabetes: a systematic review and meta-analysis. *Lancet.* 2009;373(9677):1773–1779.

7. O'Sullivan JB. The Boston Gestational Diabetes Studies: review and perspectives. In: Sutherland HW, Stowers JM, Pearson DWM (eds.), *Carbohydrate Metabolism in Pregnancy and the Newborn IV.* 1989: Springer, London. pp. 287–294.

8. Kim C, Newton KM, Knopp RH. Gestational diabetes and the incidence of type 2 diabetes: a systematic review. *Diabetes Care.* 2002;25(10):1862–1868.

9. Kim C, Tabaei BP, Burke R, et al. Missed opportunities for type 2 diabetes mellitus screening among women with a history of gestational diabetes mellitus. *Am J Public Health.* 2006;96(9):1643–1648.

10. Lauenborg J, Grarup N, Damm P, et al. Common type 2 diabetes risk gene variants associate with gestational diabetes. *J Clin Endocrinol Metab.* 2009;94(1):145–150.

11. Kc K, Shakya S, Zhang H. Gestational diabetes mellitus and macrosomia: a literature review. *Ann Nutr Metab.* 2015;66(Suppl 2):14–20.

12. Henriksen T. The macrosomic fetus: a challenge in current obstetrics. *Acta Obstet Gynecol Scand.* 2008;87(2):134–145.

13. HAPO Study Cooperative Research Group, Metzger BE, Lowe LP, et al. Hyperglycemia and adverse pregnancy outcomes. *N Engl J Med.* 2008;358(19):1991–2002.

14. Radaelli T, Lepercq J, Varastehpour A, Basu S, Catalano PM, Hauguel-De Mouzon S. Differential regulation of genes for fetoplacental lipid pathways in pregnancy with gestational and type 1 diabetes mellitus. *Am J Obstet Gynecol.* 2009;201(2):209.e1–209.e10.

15. Horvath K, Koch K, Jeitler K, et al. Effects of treatment in women with gestational diabetes mellitus: Systematic review and meta-analysis. *BMJ.* 2010;340:c1395.

16. Mitanchez D, Yzydorczyk C, Siddeek B, Boubred F, Benahmed M, Simeoni U. The offspring of the diabetic mother—short- and long-term implications. *Best Pract Res Clin Obstet Gynaecol.* 2015 Feb;29(2):256–269.

17. Reece EA. Diabetes-induced birth defects: what do we know? What can we do? *Curr Diab Rep.* 2012;12(1):24–32.

18. Correa A, Gilboa SM, Besser LM, et al. Diabetes mellitus and birth defects. *Am J Obstet Gynecol.* 2008;199(3):237.e1–237.e9.

19. Dudley DJ. Diabetic-associated stillbirth: incidence, pathophysiology, and prevention. *Obstet Gynecol Clin North Am.* 2007;34(2):293-ix.

20. Demarini S, Mimouni F, Tsang RC, Khoury J, Hertzberg V. Impact of metabolic control of diabetes during pregnancy on neonatal hypocalcemia: a randomized study. *Obstet Gynecol.* 1994;83(6):918–922.

21. Dabelea D. The predisposition to obesity and diabetes in offspring of diabetic mothers [published correction appears in *Diabetes Care.* 2007 Dec;30(12):3154]. *Diabetes Care.* 2007;30(Suppl 2):S169–S174.

22. Pettitt DJ, Nelson RG, Saad MF, Bennett PH, Knowler WC. Diabetes and obesity in the offspring of Pima Indian women with diabetes during pregnancy. *Diabetes Care.* 1993;16(1):310–314.

23. Pettitt DJ, Baird HR, Aleck KA, Bennett PH, Knowler WC. Excessive obesity in offspring of Pima Indian women with diabetes during pregnancy. *N Engl J Med.* 1983;308(5):242–245.

24. Dabelea D, Hanson RL, Lindsay RS, et al. Intrauterine exposure to diabetes conveys risks for type 2 diabetes and obesity: a study of discordant sibships. *Diabetes.* 2000;49(12):2208–2211.

25. Gillman MW, Rifas-Shiman S, Berkey CS, Field AE, Colditz GA. Maternal gestational diabetes, birth weight, and adolescent obesity. *Pediatrics.* 2003;111(3):e221–e226.

26. Pettitt DJ, Knowler WC, Bennett PH, Aleck KA, Baird HR. Obesity in offspring of diabetic Pima Indian women despite normal birth weight. *Diabetes Care.* 1987;10(1):76–80.

27. Zhang F, Xiao X, Liu D, Dong X, Sun J, Zhang X. Increased cord blood angiotensin II concentration is associated with decreased insulin sensitivity in the offspring of mothers with gestational diabetes mellitus. *J Perinatol.* 2013;33(1):9–14.

Diabetic emergencies: Diabetic ketoacidosis and hyperosmolar hyperglycemic state

SEJAL DOSHI AND HARIKRASHNA BHATT

KEY POINTS

- Pregnancy induces a relative state of insulin resistance by increasing counterregulatory hormones and maternal adiposity, which inhibit the peripheral uptake of glucose.
- Infection and medication noncompliance are the most common causes of diabetic ketoacidosis (DKA) and hyperosmolar hyperglycemic state (HHS).
- DKA is characterized by hyperglycemia, usually >250 mg/dL, ketonemia, and metabolic acidosis.

- Diagnostic features of HHS typically include serum pH >7.3, bicarbonate levels >18 mEq/L, low to absent ketonemia, profound dehydration, blood glucose >600 mg/dL, and serum osmolality ≥320 mOsm/kg. Some cases also present with an alteration in consciousness.
- Treatment of DKA and HHS requires administration of intravenous (IV) insulin, IV fluids, electrolyte repletion, and identification and treatment of precipitating factors.

EPIDEMIOLOGY

- Incidence and prevalence
  - In the general population, diabetic keto-acidosis (DKA) accounts for 8–29% of all diabetic-related hospital admissions in the United States.
  - The incidence of hospitalizations for hyper-osmolar hyperglycemic state (HHS) pales in comparison at <1%.[1,2]
  - The incidence of DKA is higher in pregnant patients at close to 9% as opposed to 3% in the nonpregnant population.
  - Multiple epidemiologic studies have reported the occurrence of DKA to be

highest in children and young adults with type I DM, whereas HHS is usually seen in the older, type II diabetic population.[3] Nevertheless, there is considerable overlap in the incidence of both disease entities among all age groups and diabetic types.
  - Analyses of the international diabetes registry databases in Germany, Austria, the United States, and England demonstrated that females were at higher risk for developing DKA compared to males.[4]
- Mortality
  - Prior to the advent of insulin therapy, the mortality rate for DKA was >90%.

DOI: 10.1201/9781003027577-8

- After the introduction of insulin, the mortality rate for DKA has declined to <2%.
- The rate of mortality in those with HHS is 10 times higher than those with DKA, ranging from 5% to 16%.[1,2]

PATHOPHYSIOLOGY

- A multitude of physiologic changes take place during pregnancy which can predispose pregnant women to both DKA and HHS.
  - These decompensated diabetic states are a consequence of insulin deficiency and increased production of counterregulatory hormones such as cortisol, placental growth hormone, placental lactogen, glucagon, leptin, and catecholamines.
  - Maternal adiposity, in addition to these hormones, acts to inhibit the peripheral uptake of glucose in the mother, promoting a state of relative insulin resistance starting from mid-gestation through the third trimester.[5]
  - Impairment in maternal insulin sensitivity contributes to the development of DKA and HHS via increased hepatic gluconeogenesis and glycogenolysis as well as reduced glucose utilization in peripheral tissues.
  - Insulin deficiency, either relative or absolute, results in breakdown of protein and lipids through stimulation of hormone-sensitive lipase. This enhancement of lipolysis causes increased free fatty acid production, which in turn leads to the production of ketone bodies, namely acetoacetate and β-hydroxybutyrate, in the liver.[6] The increased production of these acids leads to metabolic acidosis and a decrease in bicarbonate levels, which serves as the hallmark for the diagnosis of DKA.
  - Elevated levels of progesterone in pregnancy stimulate respiration and exhalation of carbon dioxide. This increase in minute ventilation induces a state of respiratory alkalosis and causes a compensatory decline in bicarbonate levels.[1,7] The altered respiratory buffering capacity in pregnancy makes this population more apt to developing DKA.
- Although the pathogenesis of HHS is similar to DKA, HHS is distinguished by the presence of more severe dehydration, smaller increases in the production of counterregulatory hormones, and enough insulin to suppress lipolysis and, therefore, ketone body production.[8]
- Precipitating factors
  - Infection and insulin noncompliance are the most common causes of DKA and HHS. Infection is the most common etiology worldwide, whereas insulin noncompliance is the most common in the United States.
  - Stress, trauma, surgery, myocardial infarction, cerebrovascular accident, pancreatitis, hyperemesis gravidarum, prolonged vomiting, gastroparesis, acromegaly, G6PD deficiency, and insulin pump failure have also been involved in the development of both DKA and HHS.[2]
  - Medications that affect glucose metabolism can lead to both DKA or HHS such as thiazides, steroids, β-blockers, atypical antipsychotics, dobutamine, or certain chemotherapeutic agents.[3] Specifically, the sodium-glucose co-transporter 2 (SGLT-2) inhibitors can lead to euglycemic DKA, with an incidence of <0.5% in type II DM and 10% in type I DM.
  - Use of illicit drugs, such as cocaine, is also an independent risk factor for the development of DKA.
  - Severe dehydration can occur due to limited access to water, immobilization, or altered thirst mechanism, leading to the development of HHS.
  - Psychological factors such as anorexia, bulimia, and depression have been reported in up to 20% of recurrent episodes of ketoacidosis in young patients.[9]
  - More than half of Hispanic or African American patients who present with DKA as the initial manifestation of diabetes have a diagnosis of type II DM. These patients with ketosis-prone type II DM develop sudden-onset impairment in insulin secretion and action, resulting in profound insulin deficiency but recover β-cell function after resolution of DKA.[10] The trigger for the sudden impairment of insulin function is unclear.
- Maternal and fetal complications
  - Maternal complications include:
    - Cerebral edema

- Acute respiratory distress syndrome
- Renal failure
- Decreased uterine perfusion
- Fetal complications include:
  - Hypoxia
  - Cardiac arrhythmias
  - Recurrent late decelerations
  - Preterm delivery
  - Brain injury and impaired brain development

the plasma volume during pregnancy increases resulting in a dilutional effect on serum glucose levels.
- Additionally, there is an increased renal loss of glucose due to increased glomerular filtration without an increase in tubular reabsorption of glucose.
- There is increased utilization of glucose by the fetus and placenta with a decrease in maternal gluconeogenesis.

DIAGNOSIS

- DKA or HHS may be the initial presentation of diabetes during pregnancy.
- Symptoms are similar to those experienced by the nonpregnant population, including:
  - Nausea, vomiting, abdominal pain, polyuria, polydipsia, poor appetite, confusion, tachycardia, hypotension, dry mucous membranes, somnolence, and coma
  - Patients can also experience Kussmaul respirations, rapid shallow breathing to compensate for the metabolic acidosis characteristically seen in DKA.[1]
- According to the American Diabetes Association, DKA is characterized by hyperglycemia, usually >250 mg/dL, ketonemia, and metabolic acidosis.
- DKA can be categorized as mild, moderate, or severe depending on the degree of alteration of mental status, the severity of acidosis and pH, and elevation in anion gap.[10]
- The diagnostic features of HHS typically include a serum pH >7.3, bicarbonate level >18 mEq/L, low to absent ketonemia, profound dehydration up to an average of 9 L, blood glucose >600 mg/dL, serum osmolality of ≥320 mOsm/kg, and sometimes an alteration in consciousness.[2,11]
- There can be a significant overlap of these aforementioned diagnostic criteria, also known as mixed-picture DKA and HHS.
- In pregnancy, DKA tends to occur at lower glucose levels and also develops more rapidly than in nonpregnant individuals.[12] Potential reasons for this are as follows:
  - In order to meet the increased circulatory needs of the placenta and maternal organs,

TREATMENT

- Management of DKA and HHS requires a multidisciplinary team of professionals involving obstetricians, endocrinologists, and anesthesiologists. Determining the cause of these emergencies through a comprehensive history and physical exam is crucial.
- IV fluids
  - Patients may have a 6- to 10-L fluid deficit, and therefore, it is imperative that these individuals have adequate large-bore IV access as well as continuous cardiac and pulse oximetry monitoring.
  - IV fluids help to reduce the levels of catecholamines and improve tissue perfusion, thereby lowering blood glucose levels and increasing the response of various cells to insulin therapy.[11]
  - Fluid options
    - Normal saline (NS) is the replacement fluid of choice and should be administered at a rate of 10–15 mL/kg/hr in the first hour.[2]
    - ½NS is appropriate if the sodium level is normal or elevated.
    - When the blood glucose drops below 250 mg/dL, dextrose should be added to the NS infusion.[2]
  - The fluid rate should be adjusted according to hemodynamic parameters such as blood pressure, urine output, or central venous pressure.
- IV Insulin
  - IV regular insulin infusion, which hinders the production of ketone bodies and lowers blood glucose concentrations, is the cornerstone of treatment for these diabetic emergencies.

- Insulin rate: Many protocols exist regarding insulin administration.
  - Insulin should be initiated at a rate of 0.1 unit/kg/hr as long as the serum potassium levels are ≥3.3 mmol/L.
  - If potassium levels are <3.3 mmol/L, insulin should be held until potassium is repleted.
  - Insulin infusion rates can increase per facility-specific protocols to slowly decrease glucose levels.
  - Insulin infusion rates can decrease to 0.05 unit/kg/hr once serum glucose reaches 250 mg/dL.[1]
- Monitoring
  - During insulin infusion, fingerstick glucose should be measured hourly for the first 6 hours and a basic metabolic panel including sodium, bicarbonate, and potassium should be measured every 2–4 hours.[11] Frequency can be decreased when glucose levels are stable and the anion gap has closed.
- Discontinuation of insulin infusion
  - Of fundamental importance is awareness of when to stop the insulin infusion, as it differs between DKA and HHS.
- Discontinuation of insulin infusion in DKA
  - The purpose of insulin infusion in DKA is not to improve the glucose levels but rather to clear the acidosis as reflected by a closed anion gap. Keeping this in mind will help avoid premature cessation of IV insulin.
  - The patient should receive a subcutaneous (SQ) injection of basal insulin at least 1 hour prior to stopping the IV insulin to minimize the risk of recurrence of the acidosis and reopening of the anion gap. The dose of basal insulin can be calculated based on any of the following strategies, with the understanding that the calculation is imperfect.
  - At least 1 hour before stopping the insulin infusion:
    - Option 1: Administer patient's home dose of basal insulin.
    - Option 2: Administer a dose of basal insulin equivalent to 50% of patient's IV insulin requirements from the prior 24 hours.
    - Option 3: Assess the average hourly rate of IV insulin over the prior 24 hours, multiply by 24, then multiply by 0.7–0.8 (70–80% of the prior 24-hour average dose) to determine the new total daily dose (TDD). 50% of this TDD should be given SQ as the total daily basal insulin at least an hour prior to stopping the insulin infusion and the other 50% should be divided into mealtime boluses of prandial insulin.
    - Option 4: Assess the average hourly rate of IV insulin over the past 6 hours (often more stable rates of insulin delivery by then), multiply by 24, then multiply by 0.7–0.8 to determine the new TDD. 50% of this TDD should be given SQ as the total daily basal insulin dose at least an hour prior to stopping the IV insulin infusion.
    - Option 5: Weight-based dosing to determine TDD for patients with type I DM is 0.3 units/kg/day; for overweight or obese patients or patients with type II DM, the dose is 0.4–0.6 units/kg/day, although patients with type II DM in the second or third trimester may require 0.7–1.0 units/kg/day.[13]
  - Insulin infusion can be discontinued in DKA once the anion gap is ≤12 and at least 1 hour after the first SQ injection of basal insulin.
- Choice of basal insulin
  - If the patient was using a basal insulin prior to admission for DKA, this basal insulin can be resumed as long as the patient is aware that insulins other than detemir and NPH have not been Food and Drug Administration (FDA)-approved for pregnancy. Little data exist to indicate that other basal insulins are harmful during pregnancy

and a change in insulin in the middle of pregnancy may worsen glucose control.
- If the patient is insulin-naive, the FDA-approved basal insulins for pregnancy include detemir and NPH.
  - NPH must be dosed twice daily once the patient is eating, with 70% of the total calculated basal dose given in the morning before breakfast and 30% of the total calculated basal dose given at supper or at bedtime.
  - Detemir may be dosed once or twice daily. If dosed twice daily, the total basal dose is split 50/50, with half given in the morning and half given in the evening.
- Stopping IV insulin infusion in HHS
  - Insulin infusion in non-DKA patients may be discontinued when the glucose levels are controlled and the patient has been adequately hydrated.
  - SQ insulin should be administered close to the timing of cessation of IV insulin.
  - Dosing of the SQ insulin follows the optional strategies listed above in the DKA section.
- Potassium repletion
  - Osmotic diuresis in the setting of DKA and HHS results in depletion of numerous electrolytes, such as potassium, magnesium, phosphate, and sodium.
  - Insulin promotes an intracellular shift of potassium, and therefore, potassium levels must be monitored frequently.
  - Typically, patients experience a total potassium deficit of 3–5 mmol/kg, but the measured serum potassium is normal or even high.[11] This is due to the shift of potassium outside of cells in the setting of increased serum osmolality and insulin deficiency seen in these decompensated diabetic states.
  - In the setting of IV fluids and insulin therapy, patients can develop life-threatening hypokalemia as these treatments promote the shift of potassium intracellularly.
  - Patients undergoing treatment for DKA and HHS with a potassium level

<5.5 mmol/L should receive potassium chloride in their maintenance IV fluids to maintain normal levels and prevent fatal arrythmias.[10]
  - If the potassium level is >5.5 mmol/L, potassium chloride should not be initially administered with IV NS.[3]
- Bicarbonate administration
  - Bicarbonate supplementation is not recommended during pregnancy as it can be harmful to the fetus and there is a lack of evidence regarding its beneficial effects.[10,11]

REFERENCES

1. Kitabchi A, Ebenezer N. Hyperglycemic Crises in Diabetes Mellitus: Diabetic Ketoacidosis and Hyperglycemic Hyperosmolar State. *Endocrinology Metabolism Clinics of North America* 35 (2006): 725–751.
2. Pasquel FJ, Umpierrez GE. Hyperosmolar Hyperglycemic State: A History Review of the Clinical Presentation, Diagnosis, and Treatment. *Diabetes Care* 37(11) (2014): 3124–3131.
3. Fayman M et al. Management of Hyperglycemic Crises: Diabetic Ketoacidosis and Hyperglycemic Hyperosmolar State. *Medical Clinics of North America* 101(3) (2017): 587–606.
4. Maahs DM et al. Rates of Diabetic Ketoacidosis: International Comparison with 49,859 Pediatric Patients with Type 1 Diabetes from England, Wales, the U.S., Austria, and Germany. *Diabetes Care* 38 (2015):1876–1882.
5. Ulla K et al. Determinants of Maternal Insulin Resistance during Pregnancy: An Updated Overview. *Journal of Diabetes Research* 2019:5320156 (2019): 1–9.
6. Barbour LA et al. Cellular Mechanisms for Insulin Resistance in Normal Pregnancy and Gestational Diabetes. *Diabetes Care* 30 (2) (2007): S112–S119.
7. LoMauro A, Aliverti A. Respiratory Physiology of Pregnancy. *Breathe* 11(4) (2015): 297–301.
8. Balasse EO, Fery F. Ketone Body Production and Disposal: Effects of Fasting, Diabetes,

and Exercise. *Diabetes Metabolism Reviews* 5 (1989): 247–270.

9. Shama R, Tareen K. Psychological Aspects of Diabetes Management: Dilemma of Diabetes Distress. *Translational Pediatrics* 6(4) (2017): 383–396.

10. Kitbachi AE et al. Hyperglycemic Crises in Adult Patients with Diabetes. *Diabetes Care* 32(7) (2009): 1335–1343.

11. Mohan M et al. Management of Diabetic Ketoacidosis in Pregnancy. *Obstetrician and Gynaecologist* 19 (2017): 55–62.

12. Chico MA et al. Normoglycemic Diabetic Ketoacidosis in Pregnancy. *Journal of Perinatology* 28(4) (2008): 310–312.

13. Alfadhli EM. Gestational Diabetes Mellitus. *Saudi Medical Journal* 36(4) 2015: 399–406.

CHAPTER 3

Thyroid

3a

Hypothyroidism

NADIA BARGHOUTHI AND VLADIMER BAKHUTASHVILI

KEY POINTS

- Hypothyroidism is defined by abnormal levels of thyroid-stimulating hormone (TSH) and free thyroxine (T4), indicating insufficient circulating thyroid hormone levels.
- Hypothyroidism poses a risk for pregnancy as well as for offspring following delivery.
- Hypothyroidism is the second most common endocrine abnormality in pregnancy after diabetes.
- Diagnosis of hypothyroidism depends upon the finding of elevated TSH, with or without a low free T4; or rarely a low or normal TSH with a low free T4 in the setting of central hypothyroidism. Trimester-specific values for thyroid hormone levels are necessary to make proper decisions regarding thyroid hormone status.
- Assessment of thyroperoxidase antibody (TPO Ab) status can help guide decision-making during pregnancy.
- Treatment involves the use of levothyroxine and achievement of a euthyroid state, with a goal TSH < 2.5 mIU/L in the first trimester and <3.0 mIU/L in the second and third trimesters.

EPIDEMIOLOGY

- The most common form of thyroid dysfunction during pregnancy is hypothyroidism.[1]
- The upper reference limit of TSH may vary among populations partially due to iodine status, the specific TSH assay used, ethnicity, geography, and BMI. By comparison, at least 3% of healthy women of childbearing age who are not pregnant have an elevated TSH, with even higher prevalence in iodine deficient areas.[2] Further details regarding specific TSH reference ranges in pregnancy can be found in the Diagnosis section of this chapter.
- Prevalence
  - The prevalence of hypothyroidism of any sort in pregnancy is generally in the range of 2–6% but, depending on the precise reference level and TSH assay used as well as the stage of pregnancy at which testing occurs, the prevalence in some studies has been reported as high as 20%.[3,4]
  - Thyroid autoantibodies may be identified in 5–15% of women during childbearing age.[5]
- Incidence
  - The incidence of overt hypothyroidism during pregnancy is approximately 0.3–0.5%.
  - Subclinical hypothyroidism affects 2–3% of pregnancies and represents up to 95% of all cases of hypothyroidism in pregnancy.
  - Isolated hypothyroxinemia affects fewer than 0.2% of pregnancies.[1,6]

DOI: 10.1201/9781003027577-10

Table 3a.1 Hypothyroidism categories

Hypothyroidism category	TSH concentration	Free T4 concentration
Overt hypothyroidism	Elevated	Low
Subclinical hypothyroidism	Elevated	Normal
Isolated hypothyroxinemia	Normal	Low
Central hypothyroidism	Low or normal	Low

- Risks to pregnancy in those with untreated hypothyroidism
  - 60% risk of fetal loss
  - 22% risk of gestational hypertension
  - Some studies have shown an increased risk of complications in subclinical hypothyroidism when compared to euthyroid pregnant women[2-4]
- Etiologies (Table 3a.1)
  - The most common cause of hypothyroidism worldwide is iodine deficiency.
  - In industrialized countries and iodine-replete areas, the leading cause is Hashimoto's disease (autoimmune thyroiditis). Autoantibodies against thyroperoxidase (TPO Ab) or thyroglobulin (Tg Ab) are found in 2–17% of pregnant women. Fifty percent of pregnant women with subclinical hypothyroidism and 80% with overt hypothyroidism have detectable levels of these antibodies.[2,7-8] Prevalence of these antibodies varies with ethnicity and, in the US population, is highest in Caucasian and Asian women and lowest in African Americans.[2]
  - Post-ablative hypothyroidism following treatment for Graves' disease (autoimmune thyrotoxicosis) or hyperfunctioning autonomous nodules (toxic multinodular goiter) is another common etiology.[6,9]
  - Other causes of hypothyroidism in pregnancy include post-thyroidectomy status, antithyroid medication use (propylthiouracil, carbimazole, and methimazole), subacute thyroiditis, postpartum thyroiditis, and hypopituitarism (central hypothyroidism).[6,10]

PATHOPHYSIOLOGY

- Thyroid size increases during pregnancy and the production of thyroid hormones, thyroxine (T4) and triiodothyronine (T3), increases by 50%.[2]

- The growing fetus does not develop adequate thyroid function until approximately 12–16 weeks gestation. Fetal neurologic development depends upon a sufficient supply of maternal thyroid hormone until well into the second trimester and the developing fetus continues to require some maternal thyroid hormone throughout gestation.[11]
- Maternal thyroid hormone levels are moderated by several factors:
  - Increased circulating human chorionic gonadotropin (hCG) is structurally similar to TSH, with a shared α-subunit and a similar β-subunit, and has some thyrotropic activity that increases circulating T4 and lowers TSH in gravid women.
  - Elevated estrogen levels lead to increased synthesis of thyroid-binding globulin (TBG), resulting in raised total T4 and T3 levels.
  - To avoid thyrotoxicosis, concurrent activation of a placental deiodinase also increases the rate of degradation of a large percentage of T4 and T3.
  - Increased urinary iodine excretion raises iodine requirements. To ensure adequate supply during pregnancy, pregnant women should increase daily iodine intake from 100 µg/day to at least 250–290 µg/day.
- Complications of untreated maternal hypothyroidism may include:
  - Fetal loss
  - Preeclampsia
  - Gestational hypertension
  - Placental abruption
  - Non-reassuring fetal heart rate tracing
  - Preterm delivery, including very preterm delivery (before 32 weeks)
  - Low birth weight
  - Increased rate of cesarean delivery
  - Perinatal morbidity and mortality
  - Postpartum hemorrhage

- Neuropsychological and cognitive impairment in the child
- Autoimmune thyroid disease, with positive TPO Ab in particular, increases complication rates in pregnancy:
  - Increased risk of miscarriage and preterm delivery
  - Progression of hypothyroidism
  - Postpartum thyroiditis
- Subclinical hypothyroidism can also be associated with adverse outcomes for both mother and offspring. In pregnancies complicated by subclinical hypothyroidism with positive TPO Ab, treatment with levothyroxine improved obstetrical outcomes but has not been proven to modify the long-term neurological development of the child.[2,5,11]

DIAGNOSIS

- Universal screening for hypothyroidism during pregnancy is not currently recommended within the healthy population.[5,11] However, physicians should screen high-risk patients prior to pregnancy and, if the TSH is >2.5 mIU/L, then repeat TSH should be obtained for confirmation. Some guidelines support aggressive screening of high-risk patients by week 9 of gestation or at the time of the first obstetrical visit.[5]
- Women at high risk for thyroid disease include[2,5,11]:
  - Prior thyroid disease
  - Symptoms of hyperthyroidism or hypothyroidism
  - Thyromegaly on physical exam
  - Family history of thyroid disorders
  - Concomitant autoimmune diseases, e.g. type I diabetes mellitus
  - History of infertility or miscarriage
- Maternal hypothyroidism is defined as a TSH elevated above the upper limit of pregnancy-specific reference ranges, which can differ between populations. When population and trimester-specific TSH reference ranges during pregnancy are not available, then reference ranges from similar patient populations should be used. If that data is not available, then a TSH upper limit of 4 mIU/L may be used.[2]
- Maternal hypothyroidism can include TSH elevations with low or normal free T4

concentrations. Isolated hypothyroxinemia, defined as a low free T4 with a normal TSH, is rare and should not be routinely treated in pregnancy unless central hypothyroidism is suspected.[2]
- Subclinical hypothyroidism is defined by an elevated TSH and normal free T4 and can be associated with adverse outcomes for both mother and offspring.[2,5]
- Women with elevated TPO Ab have higher rates of gestational complications. Therefore, if identified, these women should be screened for TSH abnormalities before pregnancy in addition to during the first and second trimesters.[5] Conversely, pregnant women with TSH levels >2.5 mIU/L should have TPO Ab status evaluated.[2]
- Interpretation of labs:
  - TSH is the lab value of choice for decision-making regarding thyroid functional status in pregnant and nonpregnant women.[2]
  - TSH can fluctuate significantly during pregnancy; therefore, consideration must be given to gestational status in evaluation of TSH results.
  - If the medical history indicates the need to use free T4 values in determining thyroid functional status during pregnancy (such as a history of central hypothyroidism), use lab trimester-specific ranges for free T4.
  - Nonpregnant total T4 ranges (5–12 mcg/dL) can be adapted in second and third trimesters by multiplying nonpregnant normal values by 1.5-fold if trimester-specific ranges are not available.[5]

TREATMENT

- Whom to treat
  - Overt hypothyroidism: Overt maternal hypothyroidism can have serious adverse effects on the fetus and treatment is indicated in these cases. Optimizing thyroid hormone levels and doses of levothyroxine in women with overt hypothyroidism should ideally occur before conception.[2,5,11]
  - Euthyroid women with positive TPO Ab: There is not sufficient evidence to recommend for or against the use of levothyroxine for preterm delivery prevention in euthyroid pregnant women or women

attempting conception who have positive TPO Ab.[2]

- Subclinical hypothyroidism: Although there is debate, the benefits of appropriate dosing of levothyroxine to achieve a euthyroid status with TSH <2.5 mIU/L may outweigh potential risks.[1,12]
- Women with infertility: There is insufficient evidence to prove that treatment of subclinical hypothyroidism improves fertility rates. However, treatment with low dose levothyroxine, 25–50 mcg per day, has minimal risks and may improve conception rates and possibly prevent worsening hypothyroidism after pregnancy is confirmed.[2] Endocrine Society guidelines suggest treating women with infertility with low dose levothyroxine to bring TSH to <2.5 mIU/L and then treatment can be discontinued if the woman does not become pregnant or postpartum.[5]
- Medication: Levothyroxine is the medication of choice for treating hypothyroidism.
- Dosing of levothyroxine:
  - Women with hypothyroidism attempting conception should be advised to contact their medical provider immediately upon suspicion of pregnancy in order to obtain TSH to determine if levothyroxine dose adjustment is indicated.
  - Women receiving levothyroxine prior to pregnancy who are euthyroid around the time of conception should increase their dose during the first 4–6 weeks gestation to 30–50% above preconception dosing. For most, this can be done by doubling their usual levothyroxine dose 2 days of the week. The increment is greater in women without residual functional thyroid tissue (e.g. RAI ablation, total thyroidectomy) than in those with residual thyroid tissue (e.g. Hashimoto's thyroiditis).[5]
  - Women receiving levothyroxine prior to pregnancy who are undertreated and still hypothyroid around the time of conception should have their levothyroxine dose adjusted based roughly on the following:

- Increase dose of levothyroxine by[5]
  - 25–50 mcg/day for serum TSH 5–10 mIU/L
  - 50–75 mcg/day for TSH 10–20 mIU/L
  - 75–100 mcg/day for TSH >20 mIU/L
- If hypothyroidism is initially diagnosed during pregnancy, start a weight-based dose of 2 mcg/kg/day with a goal to normalize thyroid function tests as soon as possible.[10] Levothyroxine dose should be titrated rapidly to reach and maintain TSH <2.5 mIU/L. TSH should be remeasured within 30–40 days and then every 4–6 weeks throughout pregnancy.
- Monitoring treatment
  - TSH is the main determinant of maternal thyroid status and should be used to guide treatment.[2,12]
  - Monitor TSH early in the first trimester and then every 4–6 weeks thereafter, continuing to adjust the dose of levothyroxine as needed to achieve TSH goals.
  - Goal TSH is <2.5 mIU/L in the first trimester and <3 mIU/L in the second and third trimesters.
    - If T4 levels are used (e.g. in those with central hypothyroidism), aim for free or total T4 levels in the upper normal reference range.
- After delivery, most hypothyroid women require a levothyroxine reduction to their prepregnancy dose. TSH should then be checked at 6 weeks postpartum.[13]

REFERENCES

1. Teng W, Shan Z, Patil-Sisodia K, Cooper DS. Hypothyroidism in pregnancy. *Lancet Diabetes Endocrinol.* 2013;1(3):228–237.
2. Alexander EK, Pearce EN, Brent GA, et al. 2017 Guidelines of the American Thyroid Association for the diagnosis and management of thyroid disease during pregnancy and the postpartum [published correction appears in *Thyroid.* 2017 Sep;27(9):1212]. *Thyroid.* 2017;27(3):315–389.
3. Ross DS. Hypothyroidism during pregnancy: Clinical manifestations, diagnosis, and

treatment [Internet]. *UpToDate*. 2020 [cited 2021 Jan 11]. Available from: https://www.uptodate.com/contents/hypothyroidism-during-pregnancy-clinical-manifestations-diagnosis-and-treatment

4. Dulek H, Vural F, Aka N, Zengin S. The prevalence of thyroid dysfunction and its relationship with perinatal outcomes in pregnant women in the third trimester. *North Clin Istanb*. 2019;6(3):267–272.

5. Vaidya B., Chan SY. Thyroid Physiology and Thyroid Diseases in Pregnancy. In: Vitti P, Hegedus L. (eds) *Thyroid Diseases: Pathogenesis, Diagnosis, and Treatment*. Springer, Cham. 2017. 674–688.

6. Dong AC, Stagnaro-Green A. Differences in diagnostic criteria mask the true prevalence of thyroid disease in pregnancy: A systematic review and meta-analysis. *Thyroid*. 2019;29(2):278–289.

7. Negro R, Stagnaro-Green A. Diagnosis and management of subclinical hypothyroidism in pregnancy. *BMJ*. 2014;349:g4929.

8. Jameson JL, DeGroot LJ, De Kretser DM, et al., eds. *Endocrinology: Adult & Pediatric*. 7th ed. Elsevier/Saunders, Philadelphia, PA. 2016.

9. Cooper DS. Antithyroid drugs. *N Engl J Med*. 2005;352(9):905–917.

10. Taylor PN, Lazarus, JH. Hypothyroidism in Pregnancy. In: Molitch M, Ioachimescu A (eds). *Pregnancy and Endocrine Disorders*. Elsevier, Philadelphia. 2019. 547–556.

11. De Groot L, Abalovich M, Alexander EK, et al. Management of thyroid dysfunction during pregnancy and postpartum: An Endocrine Society clinical practice guideline. *J Clin Endocrinol Metab*. 2012;97(8):2543–2565.

12. Practice Bulletin No. 148: Thyroid disease in pregnancy. *Obstetrics & Gynecology*. 2015;125(4):996–1005.

13. Haddow JE, Palomaki GE, Allan WC, et al. Maternal thyroid deficiency during pregnancy and subsequent neuropsychological development of the child. *N Engl J Med*. 1999;341(8):549–555.

Hyperthyroidism

JESSICA PERINI

EPIDEMIOLOGY

- Thyrotoxicosis prevalence during pregnancy in the United States ranges from 0.2 to 0.7%.[1]
- The most common cause of hyperthyroidism in pregnancy is gestational thyrotoxicosis.[2]
  - Usually transient
  - Occurs during the first trimester and usually abates by the second trimester
  - 2–3% prevalence
- Graves' disease affects approximately 0.2% of pregnancies and is the most common reason for hyperthyroidism that lasts throughout pregnancy.[3]

PATHOPHYSIOLOGY

- Definitions
  - Thyrotoxicosis
    - Excess circulating thyroid hormones from any source leading to clinically significant signs and symptoms of hypermetabolism
    - Sources of excess thyroid hormone include the patient's own thyroid gland, medications, supplements, or hydatidiform mole/molar pregnancy
  - Hyperthyroidism
    - Active production of excess thyroid hormones, thyroxine (T4) and triiodothyronine (T3), by the thyroid gland
    - The most common cause of thyrotoxicosis
- Normal physiology of pregnancy can suggest thyroid dysfunction
  - Thyroxine-binding globulin (TBG) and total T4 levels rise to a peak, frequently above the normal range, around gestational week 16 and remain elevated throughout pregnancy.
  - Total T4 and T3 increase mainly as a consequence of elevated levels of TBG, and not as an indication of elevated levels of active circulating thyroid hormone.
  - Typically, free T4 and free T3 levels do not rise above the trimester-specific range.
  - Human chorionic gonadotropin (hCG) levels rise and stimulate thyroid-stimulating hormone (TSH) receptors on the thyroid gland, increasing T4 and T3 production.

- Negative feedback by the rising thyroid hormone levels causes a decline in TSH to below normal nonpregnant range in 15% of women during the first trimester and may be below normal nonpregnant range in 5% of women without true thyroid hormone dysfunction.[4]
- Maternal complications of thyrotoxicosis[5,6]
  - Hypertension/Preeclampsia
  - Increased risk of miscarriage or premature birth
  - Thyroid storm
  - Cardiac arrhythmias or heart failure
- Fetal and neonatal complications of thyrotoxicosis
  - Incidence of fetal or neonatal hyperthyroidism is up to 5% in women with a current or past history of Graves' disease.[7]
  - Thyrotropin receptor antibodies (TRAb), thyroid-stimulating immunoglobulins (TSI), and antithyroid medications (methimazole and propylthiouracil [PTU]) cross the placenta and can affect fetal thyroid function.
  - Due to the high placental activity of type 3 deiodinase which degrades T4 and T3, maternal T4 and T3 do not significantly cross the placenta.
  - Poor outcomes include[8,9]:
    - Low birth weight
    - Fetal goiter
    - Fetal tachycardia (persistent HR > 170 bpm)
    - Intrauterine growth restriction (IUGR)
    - Fetal cardiac failure
    - Advanced bone age
    - Fetal hydrops

DIAGNOSIS

- Some signs and symptoms may mimic those seen in pregnancy
  - Feeling of warmth and/or excessive sweating
  - Heart palpitations
  - Difficulty sleeping and/or fatigue
  - Inability to gain appropriate pregnancy weight or weight loss despite adequate intake
  - Increased appetite
  - Changes in bowel habits
  - Mood changes including irritability or anxiety
  - Fine hand tremor
  - Eye findings: Dry eyes, proptosis, or exophthalmos
  - Thyromegaly/goiter
- Labs
  - Low TSH, elevated T4, elevated T3
    - Lower end of the normal range for TSH is shifted downward by approximately 0.1–0.2 mIU/L throughout pregnancy and is most pronounced during the first trimester.
    - TSH may be below the nonpregnant normal range throughout the entire first half of pregnancy without being an indication of thyrotoxicosis.[10,11]
    - If trimester-specific reference ranges are not available, the American Thyroid Association guidelines regarding thyrotoxicosis and pregnancy recommend the following:
      - First trimester: Lower end of normal range for TSH should be reduced by 0.4 mIU/L. A TSH below this is consistent with thyrotoxicosis.
      - Second and third trimesters: TSH normal range trends upward toward nonpregnant ranges. Total T4 and T3 >1.5 times normal non-pregnant range is consistent with thyrotoxicosis.
      - Elevated free T4 above trimester-specific reference ranges is consistent with thyrotoxicosis.
- Etiologies: Understanding the etiology is necessary in order to determine the appropriate treatment (Table 3b.1).
  - Gestational thyrotoxicosis
    - Most common etiology during the first trimester, occurring in 1–3% of pregnancies
    - hCG and TSH share a common α and similar β-subunits; therefore, hCG can stimulate TSH receptors on the thyroid gland, leading to overproduction of thyroid hormone
      - Incidence is higher in multiple gestation pregnancies due to greater hCG levels

Table 3b.1 Characteristic features of etiologies of thyrotoxicosis

Etiology	Characteristics
Autonomous thyroid nodule(s)	• Nodular gland on physical exam, confirmed with thyroid ultrasound • Total T3 >20 times higher than total T4 • More common in populations with known iodine deficiency • Rare in women younger than age 40
Gestational thyrotoxicosis	• First trimester • No Graves' orbitopathy • Presence of significant nausea/vomiting • Absence of TRAb and TSI
Graves' disease	• Positive TRAb or TSI • Graves' orbitopathy • Total T3 >20 times higher than total T4 • History of autoimmune disease • Abnormal thyroid labs persisting beyond first trimester
Transient thyroiditis	• Negative thyroid autoantibodies • No Graves' orbitopathy • Total T3 <20 times higher than total T4
hCG-mediated thyrotoxicosis	• Multiple gestation pregnancy • Molar pregnancy • Choriocarcinoma • Negative thyroid autoantibodies • Significantly elevated hCG levels
Iatrogenic/factitious	• Use of thyroid hormone preparations including levothyroxine, liothyronine, or desiccated thyroid hormone • Low thyroglobulin (Tg) levels

- Associated with hyperemesis gravidarum (severe nausea and vomiting with dehydration, >5% weight loss, and ketonuria)
- Resolves by gestational weeks 14–18 as hCG levels decline
- Autoimmune
  - Graves' disease
    - Second most common etiology of thyrotoxicosis in pregnancy
    - TSI binds to TSH receptors and stimulates thyroid gland overproduction of thyroid hormones. Elevated TSI levels are consistent with a diagnosis of Graves' disease
    - Elevated TRAb also indicates autoimmune thyroid disease. However, 3–5% of people with newly diagnosed Graves' disease may have negative TRAb[12,13]
  - Hashitoxicosis

- Thyroperoxidase antibodies (TPO Ab) lead to inflammation of the thyroid gland, which can trigger emission of stored thyroid hormone in an unregulated manner
- The long half-life of thyroid hormone (approximately 7 days) leads to several weeks to months of peripherally-circulating high levels of thyroid hormone, which leads to thyrotoxicosis. The thyroid gland itself, after the initial 'spill', is no longer actively producing thyroid hormone
- Thyroiditis, painless or painful
  - Passive uncontrolled release of preformed thyroid hormone into the circulation from a damaged thyroid gland
  - Due to the long half-life of thyroid hormone, thyrotoxicosis can develop

and linger for 3–6 months or more before the circulating thyroid hormone has cleared. There is no active thyroid hormone production by the thyroid gland in thyroiditis
- Hashitoxicosis is a form of painless thyroiditis
- Toxic thyroid nodule(s):
  - Unregulated overproduction of thyroid hormone by autonomously functioning nodule (toxic adenoma) or nodules (toxic multinodular goiter)
- Exogenous/Iatrogenic
  - Medications: Excess levothyroxine, amiodarone, lithium, interferon-α, PD-1 inhibitors (e.g., nivolumab), CTLA-4 inhibitors (e.g., ipilimumab)
  - Supplements: Those containing animal thyroid or high amounts of iodine
  - Iodide
  - Biotin: Not a true thyrotoxicosis Biotin interferes with some laboratory assays; therefore, the presence of biotin in a blood sample can result in spuriously low TSH or high free T4 without the presence of true thyroid hormone dysfunction
- Rare causes of thyrotoxicosis in pregnancy
  - Trophoblastic tumor
    - hCG-producing molar pregnancy or choriocarcinoma
    - Diffusely overactive thyroid as hCG stimulates overproduction of thyroid hormone from the thyroid gland
    - No eye symptoms
    - No measurable thyroid autoantibodies
    - hCG higher than expected for gestational age
  - Struma ovarii
    - Functional thyroid tissue in the ovary
    - Most often found in ovarian teratomas, rarely in mucinous or serous cystadenomas of the ovary
  - Functional thyroid cancer metastases
- TSH receptor mutation leading to hypersensitivity to normal hCG levels
- Determining etiology
  - RAI uptake and scan is a common way to determine the etiology of thyrotoxicosis

in nonpregnant individuals; however, pregnancy and breastfeeding are contraindications to both I-123 and I-131 usage. Uptake of RAI by the fetal thyroid does not start until after the 12th week of gestation; thus, exposure during the first trimester is not expected to damage fetal thyroid function. Nevertheless, there is risk of radiation exposure to the fetus and all women who could potentially be pregnant and who are being considered for RAI should have a pregnancy test and, if positive, RAI use should be avoided.[14]
- Fetal monitoring
  - Fetal and newborn testing is necessary with the presence of elevated maternal TSI or maternal hyperthyroidism.
    - Ultrasound to evaluate for fetal thyroid disease is recommended in women with TRAb >3 times the upper limit of normal or in the second half of pregnancy if there is uncontrolled maternal hyperthyroidism
  - If fetal hypothyroidism is discovered[15,16]:
    - Adjust dose of maternal antithyroid medications to minimize fetal exposure
    - Consider intra-amniotic thyroxine administration
    - Consider early delivery
  - Measure maternal TRAb levels at 30 weeks.[17] If elevated:
    - Test neonate for hyperthyroidism on day 1 of life
    - Repeat neonate testing after several days if the mother was being treated with methimazole or PTU

TREATMENT

- Treatment is indicated for overt hyperthyroidism to prevent significant maternal and fetal/neonatal complications.
- Gestational thyrotoxicosis
  - Usually mild and not associated with adverse pregnancy outcomes[18]
  - If mild, generally not treated
  - If severe and associated with hyperemesis and signs and symptoms of overt hyperthyroidism, treatment includes[19]:
    - Intravenous fluids and replacement of electrolytes

- – Anti-emetics
- – May consider β-blocker
- – Methimazole or PTU are not recommended
- Thyroiditis
  - Treatment is supportive as there is no active production of thyroid hormone by the thyroid gland.
  - β-blocker[20]
    - – Propranolol is recommended as there is minimal secretion into breast milk, and no monitoring of the infant is indicated. Dosing recommendation: 10–40 mg every 6–8 hours
    - – Reduce dose as symptoms allow
    - – Calms sympathomimetic actions of T4 and T3
    - – Slows conversion of T4 to the more active T3
    - – Extended use is discouraged due to risk of IUGR, neonatal hypoglycemia, and neonatal bradycardia
  - Hemodialysis can be considered in severe thyroiditis
- Rare disorders
  - Treatment is directed at the underlying problem if due to a rare disorder such as choriocarcinoma
- Toxic nodule(s)
  - No risk for fetal hyperthyroidism as no TRAb is present to cross the placenta
  - Usually leads to mild hyperthyroidism, so does not always require treatment during pregnancy
  - If significantly hyperthyroid, can use methimazole 5–10 mg daily but, if higher doses are needed to maintain T4 and T3 at goal, consider surgical treatment with thyroidectomy during the second trimester
- Graves' disease
  - Treatment options include observation if hyperthyroidism is mild, antithyroid drugs (ATDs) including PTU and methimazole, or surgery. See section on Graves' disease management below
  - Measurement of TRAb and TSI
    - – Indicators of autoimmune thyroid activity.
    - – If the mother has Graves' disease and is currently taking ATDs or has had previous thyroidectomy or RAI prior to pregnancy, TRAb should be measured

in the first trimester. If they are elevated, it is recommended to measure again at 18–22 weeks.
- – TRAb measurement is not indicated if there is known maternal Graves' disease, but the patient is currently euthyroid on no treatment.
- – If present, TRAb can cross the placenta and affect fetal thyroid function, especially in the second half of pregnancy and for several months after delivery.
  - – Therefore, if maternal TRAb are positive, the fetus and neonate should be monitored for thyroid dysfunction and goiter.
- – High TRAb levels >3 times the upper reference range near the time of delivery increases the risk of hyperthyroidism in the neonate.[21]
- – If maternal TRAb levels disappear while using ATDs, it may be possible to discontinue the medication.

Graves' disease management prior to conception

- Women with preexisting hyperthyroidism due to Graves' disease should defer pregnancy if possible until after thyroid hormone levels are controlled (at least two sets of thyroid function tests at least one month apart indicating normal thyroid hormone levels without changes needed in ATD dosing) to help minimize complications and adverse outcomes.[19]
- If prepregnancy hyperthyroidism requires high doses of methimazole or PTU, consider thyroidectomy or RAI ablation prior to conception.[22]
- RAI ablation
  - Contraindicated in pregnancy
  - Contraindicated in those with significant Graves' orbitopathy
  - Can lead to a rise in TRAb, which can worsen Graves' eye disease or pose a risk to fetal thyroid function
  - Pregnancy test must be performed within 48 hours prior to the administration of RAI and the patient should be advised to wait at least 6 months prior to conceiving and until after thyroid hormone levels are stable

- Some patients may require a second ablation
- Patients should expect to need levothyroxine therapy lifelong for treatment of post-ablative hypothyroidism
- Surgical resection
  - May be the better prepregnancy option in those with high TRAb levels. After surgery, TRAb levels often decline
  - Patients should expect to need levothyroxine therapy lifelong for treatment of post-surgical hypothyroidism
  - 2–5% risk of surgical complications
- Antithyroid medications
  - PTU is recommended during the first trimester and may be continued throughout pregnancy. Absolute risk of maternal hepatotoxicity is low.
    - If a woman is currently using methimazole and is planning pregnancy, she can switch to PTU prior to conception or change to PTU when pregnancy is confirmed.
  - Teratogenicity from PTU or methimazole is primarily between gestational weeks 6 and 10, thus switching to PTU or stopping any antithyroid medication in this small window may be difficult.
  - For many women planning pregnancy, initiating PTU prior to conception is the safer option.
- Stopping treatment
  - Graves' disease may be in remission pre-pregnancy, as determined by the following:
    - Dose of methimazole <5–10 mg/day or PTU <100–200 mg/day
    - Antithyroid medication has been used for at least 6 months
    - No evidence of a large goiter
    - No evidence of active Graves' eye disease
    - TRAb are not markedly elevated

Graves' disease management during pregnancy

- RAI ablation
  - Contraindicated in pregnancy
- Surgery
  - Not recommended during pregnancy. However, if hyperthyroidism is uncontrolled with medication, thyroidectomy can be performed by a high-volume surgeon during the second trimester.
  - Even in the second trimester, there is a 4.5–5.5% risk of preterm labor.
  - Consultation with a high-risk obstetrician is advised.[22]
  - Pre-operative treatment with saturated solution of potassium iodide (SSKI):
    - Use only if thyroid hormone levels are still uncontrolled in the weeks leading up to surgery.
    - Iodine has a strong effect on the fetal thyroid and can lead to hypothyroidism in the fetus.
    - It is unknown if a short course, as would be used pre-operatively, poses a risk to the fetal thyroid.
- Antithyroid medications
  - Continue antithyroid medications if there is any concern about persistent active Graves' disease or if thyroid hormone levels are uncontrolled.
  - PTU should be used during the first trimester and then, after discussion with the patient regarding risks and benefits, continued through pregnancy or switched to methimazole during the second and third trimesters.[19]
  - If switching to methimazole after the first trimester, consider the potential risk of fluctuating or transiently uncontrolled thyroid hormone levels during the transition.
  - If switching from PTU to methimazole, an unproven but generally accepted conversion is 20:1 PTU:methimazole ratio.
    - For example, if the patient is taking PTU 150 mg twice a day (or 100 mg three times a day), conversion to methimazole would be 15 mg once daily[23]
  - Adverse maternal effects of ATDs
    - Both have an approximately 5% risk of mild side effects such as allergic reaction or rash
    - Agranulocytosis 0.15%
    - Liver failure < 0.1%
      - PTU has a higher risk of maternal hepatotoxicity (1:10,000) as compared to methimazole
    - Most side effects develop in the first several months of use

- Adverse fetal effects of ATDs
  - Methimazole
    - 2–4% of fetuses exposed to methimazole during the first trimester may develop[24]:
      - Aplasia cutis
      - Choanal, esophageal, and other gut atresias
      - Omphalocele
      - Malformations of the heart, eye, or urinary tract
  - Propylthiouracil
    - Lower rates and severity of birth defects in comparison to methimazole during the first trimester
    - 2–3% of fetuses exposed to PTU may develop preauricular sinus or facial cysts or urinary tract abnormalities in males[25]
  - No significant difference between methimazole and PTU regarding placental transfer and the effect on fetal thyroid function[26]
- Consider stopping antithyroid medications during pregnancy if[22]:
  - Hyperthyroidism is not severe
  - The patient has completed at least 6 months of treatment with ATDs
  - Dose of antithyroid medication is low
  - TRAb levels are low or declining
    - Third trimester: thyroid autoimmunity often wanes and ATD doses can be decreased and sometimes stopped altogether
- If antithyroid medications are discontinued during pregnancy, thyroid hormone levels should be monitored, including TSH, free and total T4 and T3:
  - Weekly labs through first trimester
  - Monthly labs for second and third trimesters
- Other potential treatments of Graves' disease in pregnancy include cholestyramine, iodine, lithium, and perchlorate; however, none of these are currently recommended.
- Block and replace therapy
  - Using high doses of ATDs to block maternal thyroid hormone production while giving levothyroxine to replace thyroid hormone needs
  - Not recommended unless the mother has a nonfunctional thyroid gland and requires levothyroxine yet still has high TRAb levels causing fetal hyperthyroidism
- Goals of treatment with ATDs
  - Both methimazole and PTU cross the placenta and can affect the fetal thyroid more potently than the maternal thyroid, potentially leading to fetal hypothyroidism while the mother is rendered euthyroid.
  - Thus, it is recommended to use the lowest doses possible to achieve target maternal thyroid hormone levels.
  - Maternal targets
    - Total T4 and total T3 within 1.5 times the upper limit of normal nonpregnant reference ranges or free T4 just within or slightly above the trimester-specific reference range, using the lowest dose of ATD possible to reduce the risk of fetal hypothyroidism or goiter
    - Normalization of maternal TSH often indicates overtreatment with ATDs and doses should be reduced[19]
    - If there is a discrepancy between T4 and T3 levels, preference should be given to T4
- Breastfeeding and use of ATDs
  - Both PTU and methimazole are minimally secreted into breast milk
  - Recommended maximum dose of PTU is 250–300 mg/day
  - Recommended maximum dose of methimazole is 20 mg/day
  - At these doses, a risk to the thyroid of a breastfed infant is considered negligible[27]
- Postpartum thyroid dysfunction
  - Most commonly reflects an autoimmune process as the maternal immune system returns to normal after pregnancy
  - In the United States, occurs in up to 10% of pregnancies
  - Usually, thyrotoxicosis, which develops within the first 3 months postpartum is caused by thyroiditis, whereas later onset (3–13 months postpartum) is more often due to Graves' disease[28]
  - Postpartum thyroiditis
    - 4% prevalence
    - Often associated with presence of TPO Ab

- Majority resolve by one year after delivery
- Treat with β-blocker for symptom relief
- New-onset or recurrence of Graves' disease:
  - Develops 1–6 months postpartum
  - Associated with presence of TSI
  - Treat with ATDs, surgery, or RAI if not breastfeeding

REFERENCES

1. Männistö T, Mendola P, Grewal J, Xie Y, Chen Z, Laughon SK. Thyroid diseases and adverse pregnancy outcomes in a contemporary US cohort. *J Clin Endocrinol Metab.* 2013;98(7):2725–2733.
2. Labadzhyan A, Brent GA, Hershman JM, Leung AM. Thyrotoxicosis of pregnancy. *J Clin Transl Endocrinol.* 2014;1(4):140–144.
3. Cooper DS, Laurberg P. Hyperthyroidism in pregnancy. *Lancet Diabetes Endocrinol.* 2013;1(3):238–249.
4. Soldin OP, Tractenberg RE, Hollowell JG, Jonklaas J, Janicic N, Soldin SJ. Trimester-specific changes in maternal thyroid hormone, thyrotropin, and thyroglobulin concentrations during gestation: Trends and associations across trimesters in iodine sufficiency. *Thyroid.* 2004;14(12):1084–1090.
5. Burrow GN, Fisher DA, Larsen PR. Maternal and fetal thyroid function. *N Engl J Med.* 1994;331(16):1072–1078.
6. Glinoer D. The regulation of thyroid function in pregnancy: Pathways of endocrine adaptation from physiology to pathology. *Endocr Rev.* 1997;18(3):404–433.
7. Pedersen IB, Knudsen N, Perrild H, Ovesen L, Laurberg P. TSH-receptor antibody measurement for differentiation of hyperthyroidism into Graves' disease and multinodular toxic goitre: A comparison of two competitive binding assays. *Clin Endocrinol (Oxf).* 2001;55(3):381–390.
8. Tozzoli R, Bagnasco M, Giavarina D, Bizzaro N. TSH receptor autoantibody immunoassay in patients with Graves' disease: Improvement of diagnostic accuracy over different generations of methods. Systematic review and meta-analysis. *Autoimmun Rev.* 2012;12(2):107–113.
9. Marx H, Amin P, Lazarus JH. Hyperthyroidism and pregnancy. *BMJ.* 2008;336(7645):663–667.
10. Millar LK, Wing DA, Leung AS, Koonings PP, Montoro MN, Mestman JH. Low birth weight and preeclampsia in pregnancies complicated by hyperthyroidism. *Obstet Gynecol.* 1994;84(6):946–949.
11. Kriplani A, Buckshee K, Bhargava VL, Takkar D, Ammini AC. Maternal and perinatal outcome in thyrotoxicosis complicating pregnancy. *Eur J Obstet Gynecol Reprod Biol.* 1994;54(3):159–163.
12. Nguyen CT, Sasso EB, Barton L, Mestman JH. Graves' hyperthyroidism in pregnancy: A clinical review. *Clin Diabetes Endocrinol.* 2018;4:4. Published 2018 Mar 1.
13. Weetman AP. Graves' disease. *N Engl J Med.* 2000;343(17):1236–1248.
14. Polak M, Le Gac I, Vuillard E, et al. Fetal and neonatal thyroid function in relation to maternal Graves' disease. *Best Pract Res Clin Endocrinol Metab.* 2004;18(2):289–302.
15. Luton D, Le Gac I, Vuillard E, et al. Management of Graves' disease during pregnancy: The key role of fetal thyroid gland monitoring. *J Clin Endocrinol Metab.* 2005;90(11):6093–6098.
16. Abalovich M, Amino N, Barbour LA, et al. Management of thyroid dysfunction during pregnancy and postpartum: An Endocrine Society Clinical Practice Guideline [published correction appears in *J Clin Endocrinol Metab.* 2021 Jun 16;106(7):e2844]. *J Clin Endocrinol Metab.* 2007;92(8 Suppl):S1–S47.
17. Laurberg P, Nygaard B, Glinoer D, Grussendorf M, Orgiazzi J. Guidelines for TSH-receptor antibody measurements in pregnancy: Results of an evidence-based symposium organized by the European Thyroid Association. *Eur J Endocrinol.* 1998;139(6):584–586.
18. Casey BM, Dashe JS, Wells CE, McIntire DD, Leveno KJ, Cunningham FG. Subclinical hyperthyroidism and pregnancy outcomes. *Obstet Gynecol.* 2006;107(2 Pt 1):337–341.
19. Alexander EK, Pearce EN, Brent GA, et al. 2017 Guidelines of the American Thyroid Association for the diagnosis and management of thyroid disease during pregnancy

and the postpartum [published correction appears in *Thyroid.* 2017 Sep;27(9):1212]. *Thyroid.* 2017;27(3):315–389.

20. Klasco RK. 2005 REPROTOX® Database. *Truven Health Analytics*, Greenwood Village, Colorado.

21. Abeillon-du Payrat J, Chikh K, Bossard N, et al. Predictive value of maternal second-generation thyroid-binding inhibitory immunoglobulin assay for neonatal autoimmune hyperthyroidism. *Eur J Endocrinol.* 2014;171(4):451–460.

22. Ross DS, Burch HB, Cooper DS, et al. 2016 American Thyroid Association Guidelines for diagnosis and management of hyperthyroidism and other causes of thyrotoxicosis [published correction appears in *Thyroid.* 2017 Nov;27(11):1462]. *Thyroid.* 2016;26(10):1343–1421.

23. Nakamura H, Noh JY, Itoh K, Fukata S, Miyauchi A, Hamada N. Comparison of methimazole and propylthiouracil in patients with hyperthyroidism caused by Graves' disease. *J Clin Endocrinol Metab.* 2007;92(6):2157–2162.

24. Yoshihara A, Noh J, Yamaguchi T, et al. Treatment of graves' disease with antithyroid drugs in the first trimester of pregnancy and the prevalence of congenital malformation. *J Clin Endocrinol Metab.* 2012;97(7):2396–2403.

25. Andersen SL, Olsen J, Wu CS, Laurberg P. Birth defects after early pregnancy use of antithyroid drugs: A Danish nationwide study. *J Clin Endocrinol Metab.* 2013;98(11):4373–4381.

26. Mortimer RH, Cannell GR, Addison RS, Johnson LP, Roberts MS, Bernus I. Methimazole and propylthiouracil equally cross the perfused human term placental lobule. *J Clin Endocrinol Metab.* 1997;82(9):3099–3102.

27. Muller AF, Drexhage HA, Berghout A. Postpartum thyroiditis and autoimmune thyroiditis in women of childbearing age: Recent insights and consequences for antenatal and postnatal care. *Endocr Rev.* 2001;22(5):605–630.

28. Ide A, Amino N, Kang S, et al. Differentiation of postpartum Graves' thyrotoxicosis from postpartum destructive thyrotoxicosis using antithyrotropin receptor antibodies and thyroid blood flow. *Thyroid.* 2014;24(6):1027–1031.

Thyroid nodules

JENNIFER GIORDANO

KEY POINTS

- Thyroid nodules are common, occurring in up to 30% of pregnancies.
- Pregnancy is associated with an increase in the size of preexisting thyroid nodules as well as new thyroid nodule formation.
- Increased prevalence of thyroid nodules has been reported in women with a greater number of pregnancies.
- Assessment of thyroid hormone status in women with thyroid nodules is necessary for further diagnostic and therapeutic strategy.

- Clinically relevant thyroid nodules detected during pregnancy should be biopsied to determine the risk of malignancy.
- Thyroid biopsy is safe and can be performed in any trimester.
- The ultimate goal of thyroid nodule evaluation is the detection of thyroid cancer.
- Thyroid hormone medication should not be used to shrink thyroid nodules.
- Molecular markers are not recommended for evaluation of nodules.
- Use of radioactive iodine is contraindicated in pregnancy and during breastfeeding.

EPIDEMIOLOGY

- A thyroid nodule is a defined lesion in the thyroid gland described as radiologically distinct from the surrounding thyroid tissue.[1]
- Thyroid nodules are more common in women, occurring in 6.4% of women and 1.5% of men.[2]
- The prevalence of thyroid nodules largely depends on the method of screening and the population evaluated. Studies using neck ultrasonography report thyroid nodule prevalence in iodine-depleted regions to be between 3% and 30% and are correlated with increasing age and parity.[3-6] There are no studies assessing prevalence in iodine-replete areas.
- Risk factors for thyroid nodules include[7-10]:

  - Increasing age
  - Female sex
  - Iodine deficiency
  - History of head and neck radiation
- Pregnancy is correlated with development of new thyroid nodules and growth of preexisting nodules.[3,11] Up to 20% of women with a thyroid nodule detected in the first trimester of pregnancy developed another nodule before delivery.[3-5]

PATHOPHYSIOLOGY

The physiologic and hormonal changes that occur in pregnancy seem to affect thyroid nodule formation and growth. Studies have suggested potential

DOI: 10.1201/9781003027577-12

roles of iodine, human chorionic gonadotropin (hCG), estrogen, and progesterone on thyroid nodules throughout pregnancy.

- Iodine influence
  - Iodine requirements are higher in pregnant women due to an increase in maternal thyroid hormone production, increased renal iodine clearance, and fetal requirements. The American Thyroid Association (ATA) recommends 250-290 mcg of iodine daily during pregnancy and lactation. A deficient amount of iodine leading to low circulating thyroid hormones can stimulate thyroid-stimulating hormone (TSH) production and ultimately thyroid growth and enlargement of fetal and maternal thyroid tissue.[10]
- hCG
  - hCG and TSH are structurally similar. This allows hCG to activate TSH receptors, leading to an increase in thyroid hormones, thyroxine (T4) and triiodothyronine (T3), and a negative feedback and decline of TSH levels commonly seen in the first trimester of pregnancy. This TSH receptor activation can stimulate thyroid cell and nodule growth.[3]
- Estrogen and Progesterone
  - Thyroid cancer incidence is more common in women during the years between puberty and menopause suggesting the potential role of estrogen and/or progesterone in the etiology of thyroid nodule formation and tumorigenesis.
  - Estrogen and progesterone in vitro have a role in thyroid growth; however, clinical trials to date have not shown any consistent associations.
  - Estrogen (ER)-α and progesterone receptors are expressed in some thyroid tumor tissues.[11] Thyroid follicular cells in vitro are stimulated by estradiol through estrogen-dependent genomic and nongenomic signaling.[12] Progesterone has been shown to increase the mRNA expression of genes involved in thyroid cell function and proliferation.[13]

DIAGNOSIS

Initial evaluation of all patients with thyroid nodules should include history and physical exam, lab testing for TSH, and thyroid and neck ultrasound.

- History
  - Assess risk factors for malignancy
    - Significant exposure to ionizing radiation including head or neck radiation or exposure to nuclear disasters
    - Family history of benign and malignant thyroid conditions including multiple endocrine neoplasia (MEN) syndromes and predisposing genetic syndromes such as Cowden syndrome, familial adenomatous polyposis, Carney complex, and Werner syndrome
  - Symptoms
    - Voice changes
    - Dysphagia or odynophagia
    - Shortness of breath, cough, or orthopnea
    - Difficulty raising arms above the head
- Physical exam
  - Includes inspection, auscultation, and palpation of the thyroid and neck with close attention to any cervical lymphadenopathy
  - Thyroid nodules should be defined by size, location, and characteristics that raise suspicion for thyroid cancer, particularly firm, immobile nodules
  - Assess for Pemberton's sign: Facial flushing when arms are raised overhead close to the ears suggestive of vascular compromise secondary to thyromegaly
- Laboratory evaluation
  - Pregnant women with suspected thyroid nodules should have a measurement of serum TSH. Routine measurement of serum thyroglobulin or calcitonin is not recommended.[10]
  - Low TSH
    - May suggest an autonomous "hot" nodule or physiologic suppression of TSH by hCG.
    - Autonomous nodules may cause hyperthyroidism and are associated with <1% risk of malignancy, hence fine-needle aspiration (FNA) is not recommended.
    - If TSH remains suppressed beyond 16 weeks gestation, further evaluation of the thyroid nodule with radioactive iodine uptake and scan to detect possible hot nodules should be deferred until after delivery and breastfeeding.[10]

- In the postpartum setting, persistent TSH suppression should raise suspicion for Graves' disease, a toxic adenoma, or toxic multinodular goiter.
- Radioactive iodine (RAI) imaging and low TSH
  - Thyroid radionuclide scanning is useful to determine the etiology of thyrotoxicosis but is contraindicated in pregnant patients as radiation exposure to the fetus can damage the fetal thyroid gland and lead to hypothyroidism.[10]
  - In the postpartum setting, RAI scan with I-123 can be used in a breast-feeding patient as the half-life is approximately 8 hours if the nursing woman agrees to discard all milk for 48 hours.[14]
- Normal or elevated TSH
  - Some studies have shown modest shrinkage of up to 20% of nodules with suppressive doses of levothyroxine. This practice is not recommended due to the potential risks of iatrogenic thyrotoxicosis.[1,10,15]
  - Clinically relevant nodules with a normal or elevated TSH need to be further evaluated with potential biopsy.
  - Thyroid biopsy is a safe procedure and may be performed in any trimester.[16-21]
- Thyroid and neck ultrasound
  - Thyroid ultrasound remains the most accurate and safe imaging modality for detecting thyroid nodules in pregnancy.
  - Pregnancy has not been shown to modify cytology, hence the same diagnostic criteria for cytologic evaluation as in nonpregnant patients are applied.[22]
  - Thyroid nodules should be described based on their composition (solid, cystic, or mixed), echogenicity, shape, and margins. Additional findings to help guide malignancy risk (nodule which is taller compared to width, irregular margins, hypoechogenicity, microcalcifications) should be recorded.
  - A risk stratification system such as the ATA or TI-RADS should be used to assess the malignancy risk of a nodule based upon sonographic features.[1]

- Fine-needle aspiration of a thyroid nodule
  - FNA biopsy is a safe procedure during pregnancy and can be performed even if surgical intervention is not planned during pregnancy.
  - Thyroid biopsy allows for planning and expedited postpartum management.
  - Pregnancy does not seem to affect cytology specimens, however, there are only limited trials evaluating this.[23-24]
  - After thorough discussion with the patient, the decision to recommend a thyroid biopsy under ultrasound guidance is based upon the patient's risk factors for thyroid cancer, the ultrasound features of a nodule, and the presence of any suspicious lymph nodes.
  - The 2015 ATA guidelines estimate the risk of a nodule by classification into sonographic patterns each associated with a different risk of malignancy. Higher-risk nodules are biopsied at smaller sizes.
- When to biopsy
  - Biopsy is recommended at ≥1 cm if:
    - Solid and hypoechoic or with a solid hypoechoic region plus any of the following:
      - Smooth or irregular margins
      - Taller than wide on transverse view
      - Rim calcifications
      - Extrathyroidal extension
      - Microcalcifications
  - Biopsy is recommended at ≥1.5 cm if:
    - Hyperechoic or isoechoic or if solid or partially cystic with an eccentric solid region but lacking suspicious features including:
      - Microcalcifications
      - Taller than wide form
      - Irregular border
      - Extrathyroidal extension
  - Biopsy can be considered at ≥2 cm or observation with palpation and/or repeat ultrasound can be considered if a nodule is spongiform or partially spongiform and lacking suspicious features.
  - Nodules that are pure cysts, having no solid features, do not require a biopsy at any size.
  - The ATA guidelines typically do not recommend a biopsy of sub-centimeter

thyroid nodules unless associated with symptoms, pathologic lymphadenopathy, extrathyroidal extension, or a high-risk history.[1]

- Abnormal-appearing cervical lymph nodes should be targeted for biopsy.[1]

MANAGEMENT OF BENIGN AND INDETERMINATE NODULES

- Benign nodules
  - Thyroid nodules which have benign cytology (Bethesda II) or which do not meet criteria for biopsy should be managed as in nonpregnant patients with repeat ultrasound imaging in 12–24 months.[10]
  - Nodules with suspicious ultrasound changes or with benign cytology on FNA performed prior to pregnancy that demonstrate clinically significant growth during pregnancy should be evaluated for repeat biopsy or surgical resection.
- Indeterminate nodules
  - These include:
    - Atypia of undetermined significance/follicular lesion of undetermined significance (Bethesda III)
    - Suspicious for follicular neoplasm (Bethesda IV)
    - Suspicious for malignancy (Bethesda V)
  - May be followed conservatively during pregnancy
  - No prospective studies evaluating the prognosis of these nodules during pregnancy although the majority are later found to be benign[10]
  - Due to lack of evidence and concerns regarding accuracy, molecular testing is not currently recommended for evaluation of indeterminate thyroid nodules in pregnancy[10]

MANAGEMENT OF MALIGNANT NODULES

- Most cases of thyroid cancer detected during pregnancy behave in an indolent fashion. Investigations have failed to show additional harm due to the presence of thyroid cancer

during pregnancy in those who do not undergo surgery.[25-30]

- In nonpregnant adults, surgery is recommended for malignant thyroid nodules. During pregnancy, however, a conservative approach to cytologically indeterminate or malignant nodules is often considered.[27-30]
- Thyroid surgery during pregnancy is associated with higher operative and hospital risks in comparison to similar surgery in nonpregnant adults.[31]
- If malignancy is confirmed on cytology (Bethesda VI) and the patient opts for surgery, it is recommended that this be performed in the second trimester.

REFERENCES

1. Haugen BR, et al. 2015 American Thyroid Association Management guidelines for adult patients with thyroid nodules and differentiated thyroid cancer: The American Thyroid Association guidelines task force on thyroid nodules and differentiated thyroid cancer. Thyroid 2016;26:1–133.
2. Vander JB, et al. The significance of non-toxic thyroid nodules. Final report of a 15-year study of the incidence of thyroid malignancy. Ann Intern Med 1968; 69:537.
3. Glinoer D, et al. Pregnancy in patients with mild thyroid abnormalities: Maternal and neonatal repercussions. J Clin Endocrinol Metab 1991;73:421e7.
4. Struve CW, et al. Influence of frequency of previous pregnancies on the prevalence of thyroid nodules in women without clinical evidence of thyroid disease. Thyroid 1993;3:7e9.
5. Kung AW, et al. The effect of pregnancy on thyroid nodule formation. J Clin Endocrinol Metab 2002;87:1010e4.
6. Sahin SB, et al. Alterations of thyroid volume and nodular size during and after pregnancy in a severe iodine-deficient area. Clin Endocrinol (Oxford) 2014;81:762e8.
7. Gharib H. Changing concepts in the diagnosis and management of thyroid nodules. Endocrinol Metab Clin North Am 1997;26:777–800.
8. Leech JV, et al. Aberrant thyroid glands. Amer J Pathol 1928;4:481–492.

9. Rojeski MT, Gharib H. Nodular thyroid disease: Evaluation and management. New Engl J Med 1985; 313:428–436.

10. Alexander EK, et al. 2017 Guidelines of the American Thyroid Association for the diagnosis and management of thyroid disease during pregnancy and the postpartum. Thyroid 2017;27(3):315–389.

11. Sturniolo G, et al. Immunohistochemical expression of estrogen receptor-alpha and progesterone receptor in patients with papillary thyroid cancer. Eur Thyroid J 2016;5(4):224–230.

12. Derwahl M, Nicula D. Estrogen and its role in thyroid cancer. Endocr Relat Cancer. 2014;21(5):T273–T283.

13. Bertoni AP, et al. Progesterone upregulates gene expression in normal human thyroid follicular cells. Int J Endocrinol. 2015;2015:864852.

14. King JR, et al. Diagnosis and management of hyperthyroidism in pregnancy: A review. Obstet Gynecol Surv 2016;71(11):675–685.

15. Gharib H, Mazzaferri EL. Thyroxine suppressive therapy in patients with nodular thyroid disease. Ann Intern Med 1998;128:386e94.

16. Papini E, et al. Risk of malignancy in non palpable thyroid nodules: Predictive value of ultrasound and color-doppler features. J Clin Endocrinol Metab 2002;87:1941e6.

17. Belfiore A, La Rosa GL. Fine-needle aspiration biopsy of the thyroid. Endocrinol Metab Clin N Am 2001;30:361e400.

18. Oertel YC. Fine-needle aspiration and the diagnosis of thyroid cancer. Endocrinol Metab Clin N Am 1996;25:69e91.

19. Singer PA. Evaluation and management of the solitary thyroid nodule. Otolaryngol Clin N Am 1996;29:577e91.

20. Choe W, McDougall IR. Thyroid cancer in pregnant women: Diagnostic and therapeutic management. Thyroid 1994;4:433e5.

21. Hamburger JI. Thyroid nodules in pregnancy. Thyroid 1992;2:165e8.

22. Popoveniuc G, Jonklaas J. Thyroid nodules. Med Clin N Am 2012;96:329e49.

23. Tan GH, et al. Management of thyroid nodules in pregnancy. Arch Intern Med 1996;156:2317–2320.

24. Marley EF, Oertel YC. Fine-needle aspiration of thyroid lesions in 57 pregnant and postpartum women. Diagn Cytopathol 1997;16:122–125.

25. Karger S, et al. Impact of pregnancy on prevalence of goitre and nodular thyroid disease in women living in a region of borderline sufficient iodine supply. Horm Metab Res 2010;42:137–142.

26. Rosen IB, et al. Thyroid nodular disease in pregnancy: Current diagnosis and management. Clin Obstet Gynecol 1997;40:81–89.

27. Moosa M, Mazzaferri EL. Outcome of differentiated thyroid cancer diagnosed in pregnant women. J Clin Endocrinol Metab 1997;82:2862–2866.

28. Yasmeen S, et al. Thyroid cancer in pregnancy. Int J Gynaecol Obstet 2005;91:15–20.

29. Herzon FS, et al. Coexistent thyroid cancer and pregnancy. Arch Otolaryngol Head Neck Surg 1994;120:1191–1193.

30. Lee JC, et al. Papillary thyroid carcinoma in pregnancy: A variant of the disease? Ann Surg Oncol 2012;19:4210–4216.

31. Kuy S, et al. Outcomes following thyroid and parathyroid surgery in pregnant women. Arch Surg 2009;144:399–406.

Thyroid cancer

MARIA JAVAID

KEY POINTS

- Papillary thyroid cancer is the most prevalent form of thyroid cancer in pregnancy, with an excellent prognosis.
- The tumorigenesis effect of thyroid-stimulating hormone (TSH) plays a crucial role in thyroid cancer pathogenesis in pregnancy, modulated by various pregnancy hormones, with estrogen and human chorionic gonadotropin (hCG) being the significant ones.
- High-resolution ultrasound is the safest imaging modality for surveillance of thyroid cancer in pregnancy.

- Radioactive iodine is contraindicated in pregnancy.
- Surgery for differentiated thyroid cancer is usually delayed until after delivery except for aggressive forms and the safest surgical time is during the second trimester.
- Counseling regarding lactation and future pregnancies related to radioactive iodine should be discussed with the mother and family.

EPIDEMIOLOGY

- Thyroid cancer is the fifth most common cancer diagnosed in females of all ages; however, after breast cancer, it is the second most common malignancy diagnosed during pregnancy.[1-4]
- Greater than 90% of thyroid cancer cases are differentiated thyroid cancer of follicular cell origin with excellent prognosis (5-year survival rate of 98%).[2] Although pregnancy has minimal to no effect on thyroid cancer outcome, it can still lead to significant anxiety in patients due to unforeseen harm to self or fetus or stress regarding potential inability to breastfeed. A multidisciplinary team approach and psychological support are recommended.[5,6]

- Anaplastic thyroid cancer (ATC) and medullary thyroid cancer (MTC) are rare and associated with poor prognosis.
- Thyroid cancer incidence has been increasing globally, tripling from 5 to 14 per 100,000 individuals in the last 3–4 decades in the United States due to better diagnostic techniques for detecting papillary microcarcinomas, advancements in healthcare, and environmental factors.[7-10]
- Previously, prevalence in pregnancy was estimated between 12% and 43%.[11-14] A retrospective study of the California cancer registry from 1991 to 1999 described thyroid cancer prevalence in pregnancy as 14.4/100,000 cases.[4] Another retrospective population-based study in Australia from 1994 to 2008 estimated

DOI: 10.1201/9781003027577-13

thyroid and other endocrine cancer incidences in pregnancy as 17.4/100,000 pregnancies.[15] Both studies observed higher thyroid cancer rates in the postpartum period than in pregnancy, likely attributed to a delay in diagnosis.

- A female-to-male ratio of thyroid cancer is 3.1:1, which is relatively consistent worldwide.[16] This gender specification in the rate of thyroid cancer raises the concern of involvement of female reproductive factors in the etiology of thyroid cancer. Delaying pregnancy to late reproductive age favors cancer risk.[17]

PATHOPHYSIOLOGY

- Follicular lesions are usually benign in pregnancy, while malignant forms are mostly follicular variants of papillary thyroid cancer (FVPTC).[18,19]
- The pathogenesis of thyroid cancer involves multistage tumorigenesis, which begins either de novo or through activation of various protooncogenes and growth factor receptors, with influence of environmental and genetic factors. These changes lead to clonal proliferation and result in a differentiated type of thyroid carcinoma, either benign adenoma (associated with GSP and TSH receptor) or malignant neoplasms such as papillary (associated with RET/PTC, NTRK, or MET mutations) or follicular (associated with RAS).[20]
- Role of menstrual and reproductive factors
  - Higher prevalence of thyroid cancer during fertile years suggests menstrual and reproductive factor association.[7,16] A significant expression of estrogen receptor-α (ER-α) modulated by circulating estrogen and progesterone receptors (PR) on thyroid cancer cells indicates their essential role in thyroid cancer pathogenesis in pregnancy. Though a V600E mutation is noted in large ER and PR-positive tumors, there is no significant outcome difference in thyroid cancer patients.[21]
  - Estrogen also influences TSH levels resulting in increased thyroid cell proliferation.[22]
  - Progesterone shows a protective effect of enhanced thyroid growth and function through upregulation at the genetic level.[23]
  - High TSH is also associated with higher thyroid cancer risk. Both estrogen and

hCG influence TSH levels in pregnancy and, along with other placental hormones, play a significant role in thyroid cancer pathogenesis during pregnancy.[24,25]
  - A higher parity also plays a substantial role through repeated exposure to high estrogen and hCG, which leads to thyroid cell proliferation.[26]
- A meta-analysis of case-control and cohort studies evaluated the relation of reproductive factors and oral contraceptives on thyroid cancer. This study concluded that late age at menarche, increased parity, artificial menopause, and miscarriage have a risk of developing thyroid cancer, while oral contraceptives showed protective effect.[27] Overall, association of thyroid cancer with reproductive and hormonal factors is inconclusive due to variation in findings, scarcity of prospective trials, and possible recall and selection biases.[28]
- History of ionizing radiation, iodine deficiency, and previously treated toxic goiter are additional risk factors associated with an increased risk of thyroid cancer.

At the genomic level, estradiol (E2) activates estrogen receptors, ER-α and ER-β, which then enter the nucleus and modulate gene transcription. Nongenomic signaling of E2 is through activation of MAP and PI3 kinase signaling pathways by binding with membrane-bound receptor (mER). With BRAF mutation of papillary thyroid cancer (PTC), RAS mutation of follicular thyroid cancer (FTC), RET/PTC gene, chromosome rearrangement of TK receptor TRKA, E2 synergistically stimulates TK pathways (Figure 3d.1).

DIAGNOSIS

- Pregnant women with thyroid cancer are usually asymptomatic.[29]
- A good history, including childhood radiation exposure, familial syndromes, a family history of thyroid cancer, and a careful thyroid and neck examination, help establish disease status.[14,30]
- Since outcomes of differentiated thyroid cancer (DTC), including follicular and papillary thyroid cancers, in pregnant women are not different from nonpregnant females, a landmark trial suggested delaying diagnostic

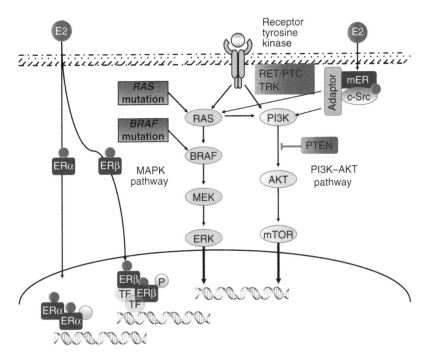

Figure 3d.1 Estrogen signaling pathway.

workup and treatment of thyroid nodules until after delivery.[29]

- Thyroid ultrasound is the recommended imaging modality in pregnancy due to no risk of radiation to fetus or mother.[31]
- Thyroid and neck ultrasound are essential for monitoring previously treated thyroid cancer, with surveillance required through pregnancy.[14]
- There are various thyroid ultrasound reporting systems with individual pros and cons. The American College of Radiology-Thyroid Imaging, Reporting and Data System (ACR-TIRADS) reporting system is highly sensitive and has excellent negative predictive value and the lowest rate of unnecessary fine-needle aspiration (FNA) biopsies in comparison to other reporting systems.[32,33]
- MRI without gadolinium is a favored imaging modality over many others in pregnancy but should be avoided unless absolutely necessary and is not superior to ultrasound in imaging of the thyroid.[34]
- RAI uptake and scan, Tc-99 pertechnetate, and other imaging modalities are contraindicated in pregnancy due to the risk of ionizing radiation exposure to the fetus.[14,35]

- As higher TSH is correlated with a higher likelihood of thyroid cancer, if a pregnant woman is noted to have an elevated TSH in the setting of a thyroid nodule, FNA may be performed more urgently.[36]
- FNA is the diagnostic modality of choice once a thyroid nodule is detected.
- A pregnant state does not alter the cellular features of a thyroid nodule, so results of FNA biopsies should be interpreted according to the recommended cytological classification and further management strategy planned according to risk stratification.[13]
- Molecular testing, which is otherwise reserved for indeterminate nodules, does not have conclusive evidence for use in pregnancy, and repeat FNA is preferred.[37]
- Thyroglobulin may be used as a tumor marker in pregnancy for monitoring of previously treated DTC.[38-40]
- Carcinoembryonic antigen (CEA) and calcitonin do not have much utility in pregnancy unless there is a strong background of familial medullary thyroid carcinoma (MTC).[41]
- Whether diagnostic or therapeutic, RAI exposure should result in immediate cessation of breastfeeding: 24 hours for diagnostic Tc-99

pertechnetate, 3 days for diagnostic I-123, and complete cessation of breastfeeding for therapeutic I-131.[42] For inadvertent exposure to I-131 during pregnancy, stable potassium iodide (KI) at a dose of 60–130 mg should be administered as a rescue agent within 12 hours if pregnancy is discovered, as KI partially blocks fetal thyroid iodine uptake.[14,43]

TREATMENT

- Treatment of thyroid cancer in pregnancy is highly dependent on the stage of pregnancy at the time of diagnosis, the overall prognosis, and outcome. Delaying surgery for DTC until after delivery has no adverse impact on prognosis and disease-specific survival.[44–46]

Surgical management

- In a study which compared DTC in pregnancy with nonpregnant women of reproductive age, 6 out of 22 pregnant women underwent thyroidectomy during pregnancy. The survival rate of pregnant patients with thyroid cancer did not differ from age-matched nonpregnant patients, indicating that thyroidectomy during pregnancy has no survival benefit but may increase fetal mortality.[47]
- A similar trial retrospectively analyzed clinical features and outcomes in 61 pregnant and 528 age-matched nonpregnant females diagnosed with DTC with 20-year follow-up. Fourteen of 61 patients underwent surgery during pregnancy and 47 delayed surgery until 12–84 months postpartum. The prognosis of thyroid cancer was the same in both groups, suggesting no harm in delaying treatment of thyroid cancer until after delivery.[29]
- Another retrospective analysis of women diagnosed with thyroid cancer during pregnancy and 1 year postpartum mirrored similar findings in favorable DTC prognosis and survival among pregnant women.[48] Though there is the recent observation of increased recurrence rates of thyroid cancer in previously treated patients, pregnancy does not affect survival.[49,50]
- The American Thyroid Association 2015 guidelines recommend surgical treatment only for aggressive types of thyroid cancer, including medullary, anaplastic, poorly-differentiated, and advanced differentiated thyroid cancer,

or if PTC diagnosed in early pregnancy shows substantial growth or metastatic cervical lymph nodes.[51]

Timing of surgical intervention

- If surgical management is indicated, it is recommended that thyroidectomy be performed in the second trimester.[37] Multiple studies have found that thyroidectomies in the second trimester had no significant maternal or fetal adverse effects.
- A study which retrospectively analyzed patients with DTC who underwent surgical resection during pregnancy and within 1 year postpartum found that there were no complications related to anesthesia or surgical procedure in either group. There were no reported miscarriages or fetal defects, although delivery of two small-for-gestational age and two large-for-gestational age infants were noted.
- Surgery in the first trimester can compromise fetal health by impairing organogenesis. In the third trimester, surgical intervention can lead to preterm labor.
- Though thyroid surgery can be performed in the second trimester with a low risk of complications, surgery for DTC can safely be delayed until after delivery.[46] A population-based cross-sectional analysis of thyroid and parathyroid surgeries in 201 pregnant females compared with 31,155 control nonpregnant females concluded that surgery during pregnancy was associated with worse clinical and economic outcomes. The maternal and fetal complication rates were 4.5% and 5.5%, respectively.[52] Currently utilized nonteratogenic surgical anesthetics were not noted to have harmful effects on fetal brain development.[53]
- To minimize surgical risk, patients should be referred for surgical intervention with only high-volume thyroid surgeons for the best surgical outcome.[54]

Monitoring

- After surgery, TSH suppression and ultrasound surveillance are the mainstay of treatment throughout the rest of the pregnancy. Reassessment of risk is performed after delivery and the need for RAI with I-131, which is otherwise contraindicated in pregnancy, is evaluated.

- In most cases, postsurgical RAI may not be necessary since 2015 ATA guidelines do not routinely recommend postsurgical RAI remnant ablation except for intermediate and high-risk patients.[51]
- For patients who defer or choose to undergo surgery during the second trimester of pregnancy, TSH levels should be maintained between 0.3 and 2.0 mIU/L.[14,36] TSH levels should be monitored every 4–6 weeks in the first and second trimesters and once during the third trimester.[19]
- Neck ultrasound should be performed every trimester.[55]
- Delay in diagnosis and treatment of thyroid cancer for more than a year can pose a worse prognosis. Poor outcome is associated with delaying treatment for more than 2 years after diagnosis.[56]

Recurrence

- As recurrence risk is low in previously disease-free patients with excellent treatment response, additional monitoring is generally not required during pregnancy.[14]
- Pregnancy may contribute to disease progression in prepregnancy persistent disease, especially with aggressive types of DTC.[57] However, the long-term effect of pregnancy on progression and recurrence is not known.[58] Although current data favor a higher rate of disease recurrence and progression during pregnancy, overall survival in patients with DTC does not seem to be greatly impacted.[59]
- For patients with previously treated thyroid cancer, a thyroglobulin level with thyroglobulin antibodies should be obtained each trimester.[57] An unexplained rise can suggest disease recurrence.
- In patients with persistent disease, levothyroxine dose should be adjusted to maintain a TSH <0.1 mIU/L indefinitely.[51,60]

Other therapies for thyroid cancer

- The use of RAI, especially therapeutic I-131, is contraindicated in pregnancy and certain precautions should be taken in the postpartum period.[14,43]
- While there are several Food and Drug Administration (FDA)-approved drugs or combinations of systemic therapy to treat advanced thyroid cancer, such as tyrosine kinase inhibitors (TKI), selective BRAF V600E kinase, and MEK1/2 kinase inhibitors, these medications are either not studied fully in pregnancy or are known to cause fetal harm. If considering initiation during pregnancy, women should be counseled about potential fetal adverse effects. If treatment is required postpartum, effective contraceptive methods are recommended.
- If painful bone metastases are present, bone remodeling agents such as zoledronic acid or denosumab can be used in the postpartum period. Given a risk for fetal harm, contraception is indicated with use of these agents.[61]
- External beam radiation, thermal or ethanol ablation, and chemoembolization can be considered for local or distant metastatic disease, but there is not enough data to ensure the safety of these therapies in pregnancy.

Counseling

- Counseling is a vital part of thyroid cancer management in pregnancy. A thorough discussion with the pregnant patient should include:
  - Prognosis of thyroid cancer diagnosed during pregnancy
  - Surgical and nonsurgical options
  - Risk of progression in previously treated thyroid cancer
  - Risk of progression due to delay in treatment
  - Risk and limitations of RAI treatment during pregnancy and with lactation
  - Postpartum treatment plan
  - Optimization with time-sensitive breastfeeding duration
- Breastfeeding can be considered for 6–8 weeks to aid in emotional bonding if RAI is deemed necessary.[62] Breastfeeding should be stopped 6 weeks to 3 months before I-131 administration to lower risk of iodine retention in breast tissue. Breastfeeding should not resume until the next pregnancy.[63]
- It is recommended to delay subsequent pregnancies for at least 6–12 months to confirm remission.[43,45,63]
- Temporary menstrual cycle disturbance is an expected side effect in the first 6–12 months

following RAI ablation.[64] Low anti-Mullerian hormone levels are noted in RAI-treated women with thyroid cancer but there is insufficient evidence to relate this with increased risk of infertility.[65]

Other forms of thyroid cancer

- Both anaplastic and medullary thyroid carcinomas are rare forms of thyroid cancer. Information regarding their management strategies in pregnancy is limited.
- Given their aggressive natures, surgery in the second trimester is recommended.
- The role of calcitonin monitoring in a pregnant female with a thyroid nodule is not well-established unless there is known multiple endocrine neoplasia-2 (MEN-2) or RET mutation or family history of MTC, though the utility is still unknown.[14,37]
- Approved TKIs for MTC (sorafenib, lenvatinib, and cabozantinib) showed teratogenicity and embryotoxicity in animal studies, but human studies are not available, leading to contraindication in pregnancy.

REFERENCES

1. Ferlay J, Colombet M, Soerjomataram I, Mathers C, Parkin DM, Piñeros M, et al. Estimating the global cancer incidence and mortality in 2018: GLOBOCAN sources and methods. Int J Cancer 2019 15;144(8):1941–1953.
2. Street W. Cancer Facts & Figures 2020. 1930;76.
3. Smith LH, Dalrymple JL, Leiserowitz GS, Danielsen B, Gilbert WM. Obstetrical deliveries associated with maternal malignancy in California, 1992 through 1997. Am J Obstet Gynecol 2001;184(7):1504–13.
4. Smith LH, Danielsen B, Allen ME, Cress R. Cancer associated with obstetric delivery: Results of linkage with the California cancer registry. Am J Obstet Gynecol 2003 Oct 1;189(4):1128–35.
5. Koren R, Wiener Y, Or K, Benbassat CA, Koren S. Thyroid disease in pregnancy: A clinical survey among endocrinologists, gynecologists, and obstetricians in Israel. Isr Med Assoc J 2018;20(3):167–71.
6. Oduncu FS, Kimmig R, Hepp H, Emmerich B. Cancer in pregnancy: Maternal-fetal conflict. J Cancer Res Clin Oncol 2003;129(3):133–46.
7. SEER 2019 database on thyroid cancer male to female ratio according to age Epidemiology.
8. Davies L, Welch HG. Increasing incidence of thyroid cancer in the United States, 1973–2002. JAMA 2006;295(18):2164–67.
9. Davies L, Welch HG. Current thyroid cancer trends in the United States. JAMA Otolaryngol Neck Surg 2014;140(4):317–22.
10. James BC, Mitchell JM, Jeon HD, Vasilottos N, Grogan RH, Aschebrook-Kilfoy B. An update in international trends in incidence rates of thyroid cancer, 1973–2007. Cancer Causes Control 2018;29(4–5):465–73.
11. Rosen IB, Walfish PG. Pregnancy as a predisposing factor in thyroid neoplasia. Arch Surg 1986;121(11):1287–90.
12. Tan GH, Gharib H, Goellner JR, Van Heerden JA, Bahn RS. Management of thyroid nodules in pregnancy. Arch Intern Med 1996;156(20):2317–20.
13. Marley EF, Oertel YC. Fine-needle aspiration of thyroid lesions in 57 pregnant and postpartum women. Diagn Cytopathol 1997;16(2):122–25.
14. Alexander EK, Pearce EN, Brent GA, Brown RS, Chen H, Dosiou C, et al. 2017 Guidelines of the American Thyroid Association for the diagnosis and management of thyroid disease during pregnancy and the postpartum. Thyroid 2017;27(3):315–89.
15. Lee YY, Roberts CL, Dobbins T, Stavrou E, Black K, Morris J, et al. Incidence and outcomes of pregnancy-associated cancer in Australia, 1994–2008: A population-based linkage study. BJOG Int J Obstet Gynaecol 2012;119(13):1572–582.
16. Kilfoy BA, Devesa SS, Ward MH, Zhang Y, Rosenberg PS, Holford TR, et al. Gender is an age-specific effect modifier for papillary cancers of the thyroid gland. Cancer Epidemiol Prev Biomark 2009;18(4):1092–100.
17. Rosen IB, Korman M, Walfish PG. Thyroid nodular disease in pregnancy: Current diagnosis and management. Clin Obstet Gynecol 1997;40(1):81–9.

18. Sclabas GM, Staerkel GA, Shapiro SE, Fornage BD, Sherman SI, Vassillopoulou-Sellin R, et al. Fine-needle aspiration of the thyroid and correlation with histopathology in a contemporary series of 240 patients. Am J Surg 2003 Dec 1;186(6):702–710.

19. Varghese SS, Varghese A, Ayshford C. Differentiated thyroid cancer and pregnancy. Indian J Surg 2014 Aug 1;76(4):293–296.

20. Moretti F, Nanni S, Pontecorvi A. Molecular pathogenesis of thyroid nodules and cancer. Best Pract Res Clin Endocrinol Metab 2000 Dec 1;14(4):517–39.

21. Vannucchi G, De Leo S, Perrino M, Rossi S, Tosi D, Cirello V, et al. Impact of estrogen and progesterone receptor expression on the clinical and molecular features of papillary thyroid cancer. Eur J Endocrinol 2015;173(1):29–36.

22. Cao Y, Wang Z, Gu J, Hu F, Qi Y, Yin Q, et al. Reproductive factors but not hormonal factors associated with thyroid cancer risk: A systematic review and meta-analysis. Biomed Res Int 2015;2015: 103515.

23. Bertoni APS, Brum IS, Hillebrand AC, Furlanetto TW. Progesterone upregulates gene expression in normal human thyroid follicular cells. Int J Endocrinol 2015;2015:864852.

24. Haymart MR, Repplinger DJ, Leverson GE, Elson DF, Sippel RS, Jaume JC, et al. Higher serum thyroid stimulating hormone level in thyroid nodule patients is associated with greater risks of differentiated thyroid cancer and advanced tumor stage. J Clin Endocrinol Metab 2008 Mar;93(3):809–14.

25. Moleti M, Sturniolo G, Di Mauro M, Russo M, Vermiglio F. Female reproductive factors and differentiated thyroid cancer. Front Endocrinol [Internet]. 2017 [cited 2021 Jan 26];8. Available from: https://www.frontiersin.org/articles/10.3389/fendo.2017.00111/full

26. Yoshimura M, Hershman JM. Thyrotropic action of human chorionic gonadotropin. Thyroid 1995;5(5):425–434.

27. Mannathazhathu AS, George PS, Sudhakaran S, Vasudevan D, Km JK, Booth C, et al. Reproductive factors and thyroid cancer risk: Meta-analysis. Head Neck. 2019;41(12):4199–208.

28. Kitahara CM, Schneider AB, Brenner AV. Thyroid Cancer [Internet]. Cancer Epidemiology and Prevention. Oxford University Press; 2017 [cited 2021 Jan 28]. Available from: https://oxford.universitypressscholarship.com/view/10.1093/oso/9780190238667.001.0001/oso-9780190238667-chapter-44

29. Moosa M, Mazzaferri EL. Outcome of differentiated thyroid cancer diagnosed in pregnant women. J Clin Endocrinol Metab. 1997;82(9):2862–866.

30. Braverman LE, Ingbar SH, Werner SC. Werner et Ingbar's the Thyroid: A Fundamental and Clinical Text. Philadelphia: Wolters Kluwer, Lippincott Williams & Wilkins; 2013.

31. Tirada N, Dreizin D, Khati NJ, Akin EA, Zeman RK. Imaging pregnant and lactating patients. Radiographics 2015;35(6):1751–765.

32. Xu T, Wu Y, Wu R-X, Zhang Y-Z, Gu J-Y, Ye X-H, et al. Validation and comparison of three newly-released thyroid imaging reporting and data systems for cancer risk determination. Endocrine 2019;64(2):299–307.

33. Mistry R, Hillyar C, Nibber A, Sooriyamoorthy T, Kumar N. Ultrasound classification of thyroid nodules: A systematic review. Cureus 2020;12(3):1–8.

34. Lum M, Tsiouris AJ. MRI safety considerations during pregnancy. Clin Imaging 2020;62:69–75.

35. Rowe CW, Murray K, Woods A, Gupta S, Smith R, Wynne K. Management of metastatic thyroid cancer in pregnancy: Risk and uncertainty. Endocrinol Diabetes Metab Case Rep 2016;2016(1):1–5.

36. McLeod DS, Watters KF, Carpenter AD, Ladenson PW, Cooper DS, Ding EL. Thyrotropin and thyroid cancer diagnosis: A systematic review and dose-response meta-analysis. J Clin Endocrinol Metab 2012;97(8):2682–692.

37. Sullivan SA. Thyroid nodules and thyroid cancer in pregnancy. Clin Obstet Gynecol 2019;62(2):365–72.

38. Nakamura S, Sakata S, Komaki T, Kojima N, Kamikubo K, Miyazaki S, et al. Serum thyroglobulin concentration in normal pregnancy. Endocrinol Jpn 1984;31(6):675–79.

39. Murray JR, Williams GR, Harrington KJ, Newbold K, Nutting CM. Rising thyroglobulin tumour marker during pregnancy in a thyroid cancer patient: No cause for alarm? Clin Endocrinol (Oxf) 2012;77(1):155–57.

40. Prpić M, Franceschi M, Romić M, Jukić T, Kusić Z. Thyroglobulin as a tumor marker in differentiated thyroid cancer—clinical considerations. Acta Clin Croat. 2018;57(3):518–26.

41. Gambardella C, Offi C, Clarizia G, Romano RM, Cozzolino I, Montella M, et al. Medullary thyroid carcinoma with double negative calcitonin and CEA: A case report and update of literature review. BMC Endocr Disord 2019 Oct 16;19(1):103.

42. Gorman CA. Radioiodine and pregnancy. Thyroid 1999 Jul 1;9(7):721–26.

43. Radiation protection of pregnant women in nuclear medicine [Internet]. IAEA; 2017 [cited 2021 Jan 28]. Available from: https://www.iaea.org/resources/rpop/health-professionals/nuclear-medicine/pregnant-women

44. Nam K-H, Yoon JH, Chang H-S, Park CS. Optimal timing of surgery in well-differentiated thyroid carcinoma detected during pregnancy. J Surg Oncol 2005;91(3):199–203.

45. De Groot L, Abalovich M, Alexander EK, Amino N. Management of thyroid dysfunction during pregnancy and postpartum: An Endocrine Society clinical practice guideline. J Clin Endocrinol Metab 2012 Aug 1;97(8):2543–565.

46. Uruno T, Shibuya H, Kitagawa W, Nagahama M, Sugino K, Ito K. Optimal timing of surgery for differentiated thyroid cancer in pregnant women. World J Surg 2014;38(3):704–8.

47. Herzon FS, Morris DM, Segal MN, Rauch G, Parnell T. Coexistent thyroid cancer and pregnancy. Arch Otolaryngol Neck Surg 1994;120(11):1191–193.

48. Yasmeen S, Cress R, Romano PS, Xing G, Berger-Chen S, Danielsen B, et al. Thyroid cancer in pregnancy. Int J Gynecol Obstet 2005;91(1):15–20.

49. Messuti I, Corvisieri S, Bardesono F, Rapa I, Giorcelli J, Pellerito R, et al. Impact of pregnancy on prognosis of differentiated thyroid cancer: clinical and molecular features. Eur J Endocrinol. 2014;170(5):659–666.

50. Vannucchi G, Perrino M, Rossi S, Colombo C, Vicentini L, Dazzi D, et al. Clinical and molecular features of differentiated thyroid cancer diagnosed during pregnancy. Eur J Endocrinol 2010;162(1):145.

51. Haugen BR, Alexander EK, Bible KC, Doherty GM, Mandel SJ, Nikiforov YE, et al. 2015 American Thyroid Association Management Guidelines for adult patients with thyroid nodules and differentiated thyroid cancer: The American Thyroid Association Guidelines Task Force on Thyroid Nodules and Differentiated Thyroid Cancer. Thyroid Off J Am Thyroid Assoc 2016 Jan;26(1):1–133.

52. Kuy S, Roman SA, Desai R, Sosa JA. Outcomes following thyroid and parathyroid surgery in pregnant women. Arch Surg 2009;144(5):399–406.

53. ACOG Committee Opinion No. 775. Nonobstetric surgery during pregnancy. Obstet Gynecol 2019 Apr;133(4):e285–86.

54. Aspinall S, Oweis D, Chadwick D. Effect of surgeons' annual operative volume on the risk of permanent Hypoparathyroidism, recurrent laryngeal nerve palsy and haematoma following thyroidectomy: Analysis of United Kingdom Registry of Endocrine and Thyroid Surgery (UKRETS). Langenbecks Arch Surg 2019;404(4):421–30.

55. Galofré JC, Riesco-Eizaguirre G, Álvarez-Escolá C. Clinical guidelines for management of thyroid nodule and cancer during pregnancy. Endocrinol Nutr Engl Ed 2014;61(3):130–38.

56. Vini L, Hyer S, Pratt B, Harmer C. Management of differentiated thyroid cancer diagnosed during pregnancy. Eur J Endocrinol 1999;140(5):404–6.

57. Hirsch D, Levy S, Tsvetov G, Weinstein R, Lifshitz A, Singer J, et al. Impact of pregnancy on outcome and prognosis of survivors of papillary thyroid cancer. Thyroid 2010;20(10):1179–185.

58. Leboeuf R, Emerick LE, Martorella AJ, Tuttle RM. Impact of pregnancy on serum

thyroglobulin and detection of recurrent disease shortly after delivery in thyroid cancer survivors. Thyroid 2007;17(6):543–47.

59. Alves GV, Santin AP, Furlanetto TW. Prognosis of thyroid cancer related to pregnancy: A systematic review. J Thyroid Res 2011;2011:1–5.

60. Pacini F, Schlumberger M, Dralle H, Elisei R, Smit JW, Wiersinga W. European consensus for the management of patients with differentiated thyroid carcinoma of the follicular epithelium. Eur J Endocrinol 2006;154(6):787–803.

61. Commissioner of the. U.S. Food and Drug Administration [Internet]. FDA. FDA; 2020 [cited 2021 Jan 30]. Available from: https://www.fda.gov/home

62. Zou J, Han L, Gao B, Wang C, Yan J, Jiang X, et al. Clinical therapy and management of differentiated thyroid cancer in pregnant women. Biomed Res 2018 Jan 25;29(1):213–17.

63. Sisson TATAT on RSJC, Freitas J, McDougall IR, Dauer LT, Hurley JR, Brierley JD, et al. Radiation safety in the treatment of patients with thyroid diseases by radioiodine 131I: practice recommendations of the American Thyroid Association. Thyroid 2011;21(4):335–46.

64. KoK -Y, Yen R-F, Lin C-L, Cheng M-F, Huang W-S, Kao C-H. Pregnancy outcome after I-131 therapy for patients with thyroid cancer. Medicine (Baltimore) [Internet]. 2016 Feb 8 [cited 2021 Jan 26];95(5). Available from: https://www.ncbi.nlm.nih.gov/pmc/articles/PMC4748924/

65. Yaish I, Azem F, Gutfeld O, Silman Z, Serebro M, Sharon O, et al. A single radioactive iodine treatment has a deleterious effect on ovarian reserve in women with thyroid cancer: Results of a prospective pilot study. Thyroid Off J Am Thyroid Assoc 2018 Apr;28(4):522–27.

Thyroid emergencies: Myxedema coma and thyroid storm

DUSHYANTHY ARASARATNAM, NADIA BARGHOUTHI,
JESSICA PERINI, AND ROBERT WEINGOLD

KEY POINTS

- Myxedema coma is rarely diagnosed in pregnancy; however, if diagnosed, treatment with intravenous glucocorticoids and levothyroxine is imperative to prevent complications to the mother and developing fetus.
- Liothyronine does not cross the placenta so its use is not recommended in pregnancy.

- Thyroid storm is diagnosed based on clinical parameters, not on the degree of abnormality of thyroid hormone laboratory values.
- Thyroid storm has a mortality rate of 10–30%, with worse outcomes in those who do not receive timely treatment.
- Myxedema coma and thyroid storm in pregnancy pose significant risk to both the pregnant woman and fetus.

MYXEDEMA COMA

Epidemiology

- While hypothyroidism is a relatively common complication of pregnancy, myxedema is exceedingly rare with fewer than 40 cases reported as of 2004.[1]
- Overt primary hypothyroidism, defined by elevated thyroid-stimulating hormone (TSH) and low thyroxine (T4), affects 0.3–0.5% of pregnancies. Subclinical hypothyroidism (elevated TSH and normal T4) affects 2–3% of pregnancies.[2]

Pathophysiology

- Myxedema coma occurs as a result of longstanding undiagnosed or untreated hypothyroidism that is precipitated by an acute insult.[3] The action of thyroid hormones is mediated by their binding to nuclear receptors, the absence of which has profound effects on all systems of the body.[4]
- Decreased T4 leads to a drop in serum and intracellular triiodothyronine (T3), resulting in several metabolic consequences. These include[3,4]:
  - Decreased thermogenesis
  - Decreased sensitivity to adrenergic stimuli
  - Increased antidiuretic hormone (ADH) secretion and renal hypoperfusion
  - Decreased central nervous system sensitivity to hypercapnia and hypoxia with respiratory muscle weakness
  - Slowing of central nervous system function

DOI: 10.1201/9781003027577-14

- The pathophysiological hallmark of this disease is diminished ventilatory drive to hypoxia and hypercapnia, leading to alveolar hypoventilation.[3] Pregnant women are at greater risk of becoming hypoxic due to increased maternal oxygen consumption and lower oxygen reserves due to lower functional residual capacity.[5] Hypoxia may be exacerbated by submucosal edema of the upper airways, seen in both hypothyroidism and pregnancy, and superimposed pneumonia, pericardial and pleural effusions, and ascites seen in hypothyroidism.[3,4] Despite diaphragm displacement by the gravid uterus, respiratory muscle strength in pregnancy is critical to maintaining the increase in tidal volume and minute ventilation.[6] Respiratory muscle weakness due to hypothyroid myopathy interferes with the normal physiology of respiratory function.[3]
- Major cardiovascular changes in pregnancy include increased plasma blood volume, increased cardiac output, and a reduction in systemic vascular resistance. These changes are important to meet increasing metabolic demands of the mother and fetus and tolerate acute blood loss that occurs with childbirth.[7] Bradycardia, cardiac enlargement, and depressed cardiac contractility are the most common cardiac findings in severe hypothyroidism. Increased α-adrenergic responsiveness and reduced β-cell receptors as well as changed coupling with adenylyl cyclase in hypothyroidism lead to these clinical features.[3]
- Hypotension and shock with a concomitant reduction in blood volume of up to 20% can occur with myxedema coma.[3] This has implications in pregnancy where the total blood volume peaks at 40% greater than baseline and smaller increases in maternal plasma blood volume are associated with intrauterine growth restriction (IUGR) and poor fetal outcomes.[7] In myxedema, the increase in maternal red cell mass typically seen in pregnancy is blunted due to a reduction in erythropoietin production, leading to a decline in red cell production and fall in hematocrit of approximately 30%.[3,7]
- Diastolic hypertension has been observed due to the decreased β-cell receptor responsiveness resulting in unopposed α-adrenergic stimuli.
- Pericardial effusion is often seen in myxedema.[3]

- Clearance of ADH is increased in the placenta, which produces cysteine aminopeptidase with vasopressinase and oxytocinase activity. Although overall ADH levels are unchanged, the increased clearance of ADH may lead to transient diabetes insipidus of pregnancy.[5] Conversely, in myxedema, excessive ADH secretion and an inability to excrete free water can lead to hyponatremia.[4] Decreased renal perfusion can lead to increased free water retention. In addition, thyroid hormone effects on Na/K/ATPase activity may lead to reduced sodium resorption in the renal tubule, contributing to hyponatremia.

Diagnosis

- The diagnosis of myxedema coma is made with the confirmation of a biochemical profile consistent with hypothyroidism and corresponding clinical manifestations.[8]
- The clinical presentation of hypothyroidism in pregnancy is similar to that of nonpregnant individuals, with symptoms including constipation, cold intolerance, cool, dry skin, coarse hair, irritability, and inability to concentrate.[9] Macroglossia, voice hoarseness, and periorbital edema are signs of gross hypothyroidism and, in combination with hypothermia, hypotension, hypoventilation, hyponatremia, and bradycardia, are characteristic of myxedema and should prompt immediate investigation.[9]
- The biochemical diagnosis of primary hypothyroidism can be made with an elevated TSH in association with a low serum free T4. This is supported by positive thyroperoxidase antibodies (TPO Ab) in a patient who has not had radioactive iodine therapy or a thyroidectomy.[9] TSH is the test of choice in pregnancy, although evaluation requires the use of trimester-specific reference ranges to avoid underestimating the incidence of hypothyroidism. Total T4 and T3 levels increase in early pregnancy and plateau in the second trimester. Increased thyroid-binding globulin (TBG) and decreased albumin may confound total T4 measurements in pregnancy.[6]
- Determining the etiology of hypothyroidism is important, specifically in patients

with TSH receptor-blocking antibodies, as these can cross the placenta and lead to fetal hypothyroidism.[6]

Treatment

- The primary objectives in treatment of myxedema in pregnancy are restoration of normal thyroid hormone levels, correction of any underlying electrolyte abnormalities, and identification and treatment of underlying conditions.
- Pregnant women require larger doses of levothyroxine due to the rapid rise in TBG, increased placental transport and metabolism of maternal T4, and increased distribution volume of thyroid hormones.
- The full replacement dose in pregnancy is 2–2.4 mcg/kg/day. In acute management of severe hypothyroidism, rapid normalization of thyroid hormone levels may require treatment with intravenous levothyroxine at twice the estimated final replacement dose.[2]
- Hypothyroidism may be accompanied by previously undiagnosed adrenal insufficiency. In myxedema, supportive therapy and corticosteroids are administered prior to the first dose of levothyroxine to avoid precipitation of an adrenal crisis. A baseline cortisol level should be obtained followed by administration of 50–100 mg of intravenous hydrocortisone every 6–8 hours until the baseline cortisol level is known, then titrated accordingly.
- Supportive therapy may include warming, intravenous fluids, electrolyte replacement, cardiac monitoring with inotropic supportive therapy, and endotracheal intubation and mechanical ventilation if necessary.
- In pregnancy, 300–500 mcg of intravenous levothyroxine should be administered followed by a daily intravenous dose of 75–100 mcg until the patient can safely take oral medications.
- Cardiac output, blood pressure, temperature, and mental status typically improve within the first 24 hours. Free T4 levels should be monitored daily and are expected to rise within the first 1–2 days of treatment.
- Liothyronine does not cross the placenta, therefore AACE/ATA guidelines do not recommend combination T4/T3 therapy in pregnant women.[10]

THYROID STORM

Epidemiology

- Hyperthyroidism affects roughly 0.4% of pregnancies.
- Approximately 1–2% of pregnant women with hyperthyroidism will experience thyroid storm during pregnancy.[11,12] Thyroid storm occurs in 3.5% of pregnant patients with thyrotoxicosis. Many of these cases occur in patients without prior treatment of hyperthyroidism.[13]
- Women with hyperthyroidism are significantly more likely to develop thyroid storm while pregnant than when not pregnant.[14]

Pathophysiology

- Thyrotoxicosis (presence of excess thyroid hormone) in pregnancy, as indicated by low TSH and elevated T4 and T3, can arise from various sources (see Chapter 3b).
  - Graves' disease: Endogenous active overproduction of thyroid hormone (hyperthyroidism), identified during pregnancy by elevated thyrotropin receptor antibodies (TRAb) or thyroid-stimulating immunoglobulins (TSI)
  - Toxic adenoma or multinodular goiter: Endogenous overproduction of thyroid hormone from nodule(s)
  - Acute thyroiditis: Sudden release of preformed thyroid hormone
- During pregnancy, the typical symptoms of thyrotoxicosis (see Chapter 3b) may acutely worsen with sudden decompensation in clinical status and development of thyroid storm. This is often triggered by an inciting event such as a viral illness, trauma, or excess iodine exposure.
- Decompensated thyrotoxicosis in pregnancy can lead to a high risk of heart failure and death if left untreated.[15]

Diagnosis

- In pregnant women with known hyperthyroidism and acute worsening of signs and symptoms typically associated with excess circulating thyroid hormone, evaluation should include:

- Lab tests for TSH, total and free T4, and total T3 for biochemical confirmation of hyperthyroidism
- Thyroid hormone levels in pregnancy must be interpreted according to pregnancy-specific reference ranges[11]
  - In first trimester, TSH is commonly low secondary to elevated hCG and total T4 levels may be above normal.
  - In second and third trimesters, TSH and free T4 in nonhyperthyroid women are typically within normal range and total T4 may be slightly above normal nonpregnant reference range.
- History to identify potential reasons for acute worsening of thyroid clinical status
  - Labor, parturition, infection, physical trauma, trauma to the thyroid gland, recent iodinated contrast studies, surgery, ingestion of large sources of iodine (kelp, supplements, amiodarone), ingestion of excess exogenous thyroid hormone (levothyroxine, desiccated thyroid preparations), other
- Physical exam to identify possible goiter, proptosis, tremor, tachycardia, hyperthermia
- Additional studies[15]:
  - TRAb and TSI if Graves' is suspected
  - Thyroid ultrasound to detect nodules
  - Radioactive iodine is contraindicated in pregnancy, thus thyroid scintigraphy should not be performed
- If thyroid storm is suspected based on labs indicating hyperthyroidism, fever, mental status changes, cardiac dysfunction, or other clinical features, our group uses the Burch-Wartofsky scoring system to classify a patient's risk of thyroid storm. This system evaluates risk based on degrees of[15]:
  - Thermoregulatory dysfunction, with higher body temperatures imparting a higher score
  - Cardiovascular dysfunction, with higher heart rates imparting a higher score
  - Heart failure, based on levels of peripheral and pulmonary edema
  - Central nervous system dysfunction, determined by levels of alertness, orientation, and agitation

- Hepatic and gastrointestinal dysfunction, with higher scores appointed for jaundice
- Scoring (Table 3e.1)[16]:
  - A total score >44 indicates that thyroid storm is highly likely
  - A total score of 25–44 is supportive of a diagnosis of thyroid storm
  - A total score <25 indicates that thyroid storm is unlikely
- It is important to note that the likelihood of thyroid storm in any given patient, based on this scoring system, is not a reflection of the degree of abnormality of the labs that indicate hyperthyroidism; rather, the likelihood of storm, in a person with any degree of low TSH and elevated T4 and/or T3, is determined based on clinical signs and symptoms.

Treatment

- Manage patient in the intensive care unit
- β-blocker[11,15]
  - Helps control heart rate and other symptoms of adrenergic excess
  - Propranolol is generally preferred
    - Slows peripheral conversion of T4 to the more active T3
    - Dosing: 40–80 mg orally every 4–6 hours
  - Titrate to pulse, blood pressure, and symptoms
  - If concern for heart failure, consider the calcium channel blocker, diltiazem
- Antithyroid medications[11,15]
  - Inhibit production of thyroid hormone by thyroid gland
  - Use propylthiouracil (PTU) if in first trimester of pregnancy
  - Use methimazole or PTU if in second or third trimester of pregnancy
  - PTU generally preferred
    - Slows peripheral conversion of T4 to the more active T3
    - Dosing: 200 mg orally every 4 hours
  - If using methimazole, dosing: 20 mg orally every 4–6 hours
- Saturated solution of potassium iodide (SSKI) or Lugol's solution[11,15]
  - Blocks release of T4 and T3 from thyroid gland

Table 3e.1 Scoring for thyroid storm

Thermoregulatory dysfunction		Cardiovascular dysfunction		Heart failure	
Temperature (°C/°F)	Points	HR (BPM)	Points	Symptoms	Points
37.2–37.7/99–99.9	5	99–109	5	Mild: Pedal edema	5
37.8–38.2/100–100.9	10	110–119	10	Moderate: Bibasilar rales	10
38.3–38.8/101–101.9	15	120–129	15	Severe: Pulmonary edema	15
38.9–39.4/102–102.9	20	130–139	20		
39.5–39.9/103–103.9	25	>139	25		
>39.9/>103.9	30	Atrial fibrillation	10		

Central Nervous System dysfunction		Hepatic-Gastrointestinal dysfunction		Precipitating event	
Symptoms	Points	Symptoms	Points	Symptoms	Points
Mild: Agitation	10	Moderate: • Diarrhea • Nausea/Vomiting • Abdominal pain	10	No	0
Moderate: • Delirium • Psychosis • Extreme lethargy	20	Severe: Unexplained jaundice	20	Yes	10
Severe: • Seizures • Coma	30				

Source: Adapted from Burch-Wartofsky.

- Do not give until at least one hour after PTU or methimazole has been administered
- Dosing of SSKI: 50 mg iodide/drop solution, 5 drops orally every 6 hours
- Dosing of Lugol's: 6.25 mg iodide/iodine per drop, 10 drops orally three times daily
- Glucocorticoids
  - Provide hemodynamic support in case of undiagnosed underlying adrenal insufficiency
  - Slow peripheral conversion of T4 to the more active T3
  - Impair autoimmune process of Graves' disease
  - Dosing
    - Hydrocortisone 50–100 mg IV every 6–8 hours *or*
    - Dexamethasone 2 mg IV every 6 hours
  - Measure cortisol prior to administration of glucocorticoids to inform later decisions regarding safety of stopping the steroid
- Bile acid sequestrants
  - Impair enterohepatic recycling of thyroid hormones
  - Dosing: Cholestyramine 4 g orally four times daily
- Surgery
  - Total thyroidectomy may be considered if the patient is intolerant of or has contraindications to use of antithyroid medications.
- Plasmapheresis[17]
  - Clears immune particles and thyroid hormone
  - Can help prepare thyrotoxic patients for surgery

- May be considered if the patient is intolerant of or has contraindications to use of antithyroid medications and/or if surgery cannot be safely performed at the time. While guidelines do not specifically address plasmapheresis for treatment of hyperthyroidism in pregnancy, there are case reports indicating that plasmapheresis may help thyrotoxic pregnant women who were unable to use antithyroid medications[18,19]

REFERENCES

1. Turhan NO, Koçkar MC, Inegöl I. Myxedematous coma in a laboring woman suggested a pre-eclamptic coma: A case report. *Acta Obstet Gynecol Scand.* 2004;83(11):1089–1091.

2. Sahay RK, Nagesh VS. Hypothyroidism in pregnancy. *Indian J Endocrinol Metab.* 2012;16(3):364–370.

3. Donangelo I, Braunstein GD. Myxedema coma. In: Loriaux L (ed.). Endocrine Emergencies. Totowa, NJ: Humana Press; 2014 [cited 2021 Jun 3]. pp. 99–108. Available from: http://link.springer.com/10.1007/978-1-62703-697-9_10

4. Sarlis NJ, Gourgiotis L. Thyroid emergencies. *Rev Endocr Metab Disord.* 2003;4(2):129–136.

5. Tan EK, Tan EL. Alterations in physiology and anatomy during pregnancy. *Best Pract Res Clin Obstet Gynaecol.* 2013;27(6):791–802.

6. Cignini P, Cafà EV, Giorlandino C, Capriglione S, Spata A, Dugo N. Thyroid physiology and common diseases in pregnancy: Review of literature. *J Prenat Med.* 2012;6(4):64–71.

7. Hegewald MJ, Crapo RO. Respiratory physiology in pregnancy. *Clin Chest Med.* 2011;32(1):1–13.

8. Leung AM. Thyroid emergencies. *J Infus Nurs.* 2016;39(5):281–286.

9. Holmgren C, Belfort MA. Thyroid and adrenal emergencies in pregnancy. *Expert Rev Obstet Gynecol.* 2007;2(3):387–394.

10. Jonklaas J, Bianco AC, Bauer AJ, et al. Guidelines for the treatment of hypothyroidism: Prepared by the American Thyroid Association Task Force on thyroid hormone replacement. *Thyroid.* 2014;24(12):1670–1751.

11. American College of Obstetrics and Gynecology. ACOG practice bulletin. Thyroid disease in pregnancy. Number 37, August 2002. American College of Obstetrics and Gynecology. *Int J Gynaecol Obstet.* 2002;79(2):171–180.

12. Sorah K, Alderson TL. Hyperthyroidism in pregnancy. StatPearls. Treasure Island, FL: StatPearls Publishing; June 4, 2021.

13. Davis LE, Lucas MJ, Hankins GD, Roark ML, Cunningham FG. Thyrotoxicosis complicating pregnancy. *Am J Obstet Gynecol.* 1989;160(1):63–70.

14. Ma Y, Li H, Liu J, Lin X, Liu H. Impending thyroid storm in a pregnant woman with undiagnosed hyperthyroidism: A case report and literature review. *Medicine (Baltimore).* 2018;97(3):e9606.

15. Alexander EK, Pearce EN, Brent GA, et al. 2017 Guidelines of the American Thyroid Association for the diagnosis and management of thyroid disease during pregnancy and the postpartum [published correction appears in Thyroid. 2017 Sep;27(9):1212]. *Thyroid.* 2017;27(3):315–389.

16. Burch HB, Wartofsky L. Life-threatening thyrotoxicosis: Thyroid storm. *Endocrinol Metab Clin North Am.* 1993;22(2):263–277.

17. Vyas AA et al. Successful treatment of thyroid storm with plasmapheresis in a patient with methimazole-induced agranulocytosis. *Endocr Pract.* 2010;16(4):673.

18. Bilir BE et al. Effectiveness of preoperative plasmapheresis in a pregnancy complicated by hyperthyroidism and antithyroid drug-associated angioedema. *Gynecol Endocrinol.* 2013;29(5):508–510.

19. Horani MH et al. SUN-509 plasmapheresis treatment of thyrotoxicosis in pregnancy for preparation of thyroidectomy. *J Endocr Soc.* 2020 May 8;4(Suppl 1):SUN-509.

CHAPTER 4

Adrenal

4a

Adrenal incidental adenomas

JENNIFER S. TURNER

KEY POINTS

- An adrenal incidental adenoma, often called adrenal incidentaloma, is an asymptomatic adrenal lesion discovered when a patient is undergoing radiologic evaluation for another issue unrelated to adrenal disease.[1–3]
- When an adrenal incidentaloma is found, evaluation should include hormone measurements for excess cortisol to rule out Cushing's syndrome, metanephrines and catecholamines to rule out pheochromocytoma, and, if the patient has hypertension, aldosterone and renin to rule out primary hyperaldosteronism.

- Evaluation of incidental adrenal adenomas for the development of excess hormone function should occur periodically over the patient's lifetime.
- Hyperfunctioning or large (≥4 cm) adrenal masses can be surgically resected in the second trimester of pregnancy.
- Adrenal gland biopsy is not recommended. However, if a biopsy is necessary, pheochromocytoma must be ruled out prior to the procedure.
- Adrenal biopsy cannot differentiate adrenal adenoma from adrenocortical carcinoma.

EPIDEMIOLOGY

- The incidence of adrenal incidentalomas is increasing with more frequent use of abdominal computed tomography (CT) and magnetic resonance imaging (MRI), as well as with improvements in imaging quality.[4]
- As imaging studies are rarely performed in pregnancy, the incidence of adrenal incidental adenomas diagnosed during pregnancy is low, with exact numbers being unknown due to the paucity of data.[5,6]
- The importance of timely identification, evaluation, and management of adrenal disease in pregnancy cannot be overstated, given the potential morbidity and mortality in both the mother and fetus.[7]

- The mean prevalence of adrenal incidentalomas in an autopsy series in 23 studies was 3% and the mean prevalence of adrenal incidentalomas discovered by CT in 13 studies was 1.9%.[5]
- The prevalence of adrenal adenomas increases with age and there is no difference in prevalence between males and females in autopsy studies.[5]

PATHOPHYSIOLOGY

- Cell types
  - Adrenal incidentalomas can arise from the adrenal cortex, adrenal medulla, or as metastatic disease from an extra-adrenal cancer.

DOI: 10.1201/9781003027577-16

- Tumors arising from the adrenal cortex include nonfunctional adrenocortical adenomas, cortisol-producing adenomas, aldosterone-producing adenomas, and adrenocortical carcinoma.
- A tumor arising from the adrenal medulla is a pheochromocytoma.[5]
- The most common etiology of an adrenal incidentaloma is a benign, non-hypersecreting adrenocortical adenoma.[8]

DIAGNOSIS

- The two questions which should be answered when an adrenal incidentaloma is discovered in pregnant or nonpregnant patients are:
  - Is the mass associated with hormone hypersecretion?
    - This is determined by biochemical evaluation, discussed in detail in other chapters (see Chapters 4b–4d).
  - Is the mass benign or malignant?
    - This is difficult to determine exclusively by imaging, but radiographic findings can raise or lower suspicion.
    - Radiographic features concerning for potential malignancy include:
      - Size ≥4 cm
      - Heterogenous content
      - Hounsfield units ≥10 on noncontrasted CT
      - CT adrenal protocol showing absolute contrast washout at 15 minutes ≤60% or relative washout ≤40%[9]
    - MRI without gadolinium is the imaging modality of choice in pregnancy to avoid unnecessary radiation exposure to the fetus.
    - Adrenocortical carcinoma is discussed in detail in Chapter 4e.

TREATMENT

- Treatment of adrenal incidentalomas in pregnancy depends on the functional status of the adenoma as well as its malignant potential (see Chapters 4b–4e for further details regarding the diagnosis and management of pheochromocytoma, Cushing's syndrome, primary hyperaldosteronism, and adrenocortical carcinoma).
- Functional incidentalomas usually require surgery regardless of size and any mass ≥4 cm should undergo resection. However, no surgery should be performed until pheochromocytoma has been ruled out.

REFERENCES

1. Zeiger MA, Siegelman SS, Hamrahian AH. Medical and surgical evaluation and treatment of adrenal incidentalomas. J Clin Endocrinol Metab. 2011;96(7):2004–2015.
2. Zeiger MA, Thompson GB, Duh QY, et al. The American Association of Clinical Endocrinologists and American Association of Endocrine Surgeons medical guidelines for the management of adrenal incidentalomas. Endocr Pract. 2009;15(Suppl 1):1–20.
3. Fassnacht M, Arlt W, Bancos I, et al. Management of adrenal incidentalomas: European Society of Endocrinology Clinical Practice Guideline in collaboration with the European Network for the Study of Adrenal Tumors. Eur J Endocrinol. 2016;175(2):G1–34.
4. Brunt LM, Moley JF. Adrenal incidentaloma. World J Surg. 2001;25(7):905–913.
5. Sherlock M, Scarsbrook A, Abbas A, et al. Adrenal incidentaloma. Endocr Rev. 2020 April 8 [cited 2020 June 29]. doi:10.1210/endrev/bnaa008
6. Fallo F, Pezzi Z, Sonino N, et al. Adrenal incidentaloma in pregnancy: Clinical, molecular and immunohistochemical findings. J Endocrinol Invest. 2005;28(5):459–463.
7. Kamoun M, Mnif MF, Charfi N, et al. Adrenal diseases during pregnancy: Pathophysiology, diagnosis and management strategies. Am J Med Sci. 2014;347(1):64–73.
8. Young Jr WF. The incidentally discovered adrenal mass. N Engl J Med. 2007;356: 601–610.
9. Vaidya A, Hamrahian A, Bancos I, et al. The evaluation of incidentally discovered adrenal masses. Endocr Pract. 2019;25(2):178–192.

4b

Pheochromocytoma

JENNIFER S. TURNER

KEY POINTS

- Pheochromocytomas and paragangliomas (PPGLs) are neuroendocrine tumors that secrete catecholamines.
- These tumors are uncommon in pregnancy.
- PPGLs may present similarly to pregnancy-related hypertension.

- If untreated, PPGLs can increase morbidity and mortality to the mother and fetus.
- Alpha blockade is the first step in treatment of PPGLs in pregnancy.
- Timing of surgery for PPGLs during pregnancy depends upon gestational age and location of the tumor.

EPIDEMIOLOGY

- Of all chromaffin cell tumors, 80–85% are pheochromocytomas and 15–20% are paragangliomas.[1]
- The prevalence of PPGLs in patients with hypertension is between 0.2% and 0.6%.
- The prevalence of PPGLs in those discovered to have an adrenal incidentaloma is around 5%.
- The incidence of PPGLs in pregnancy is estimated at 1 in 15,000–54,000.[1,2]
- As in nonpregnant individuals, most cases are sporadic and unilateral; however, other cases can be part of an inherited disorder. All pregnant patients diagnosed with PPGL should undergo genetic testing as one study found that germline mutations were identified in 30% of women diagnosed during pregnancy.[3,4]

PATHOPHYSIOLOGY

- Pheochromocytomas are neuroendocrine tumors that arise from chromaffin cells in the adrenal medulla while paragangliomas are neuroendocrine tumors that arise from extra-adrenal chromaffin cells of the sympathetic ganglia present in the thorax, abdomen, and pelvis.[1]
- PPGLs secrete excess catecholamines. Catecholamines do not affect the fetus directly due to presence of enzymes in the placenta called catechol-O-methyltransferase (COMT) and monoamine oxidase (MAO) which deactivate them.
- Maternal catecholamine excess leads to negative downstream effects on the fetus due to maternal hypertension.[2,3,5] Maternal hypertension may cause increased constriction in the uteroplacental circulation leading to uteroplacental insufficiency and the potential for compromised fetal growth and increased risk of fetal mortality.[3,5]

DIAGNOSIS

- Signs and symptoms of PPGL can include:
  - Sustained or paroxysmal hypertension
  - Hyperhidrosis

DOI: 10.1201/9781003027577-17

- Tachycardia and palpitations
- Headaches
- Pallor
- Abdominal pain and/or emesis
- Anxiety
- Dyspnea and/or chest pain
- Although some patients may have minimal or no complaints, the most common signs and symptoms of excess catecholamines in pregnancy are hypertension, palpitations, headaches, and diaphoresis.[6]
- Rare but serious presentations of PPGL are heart failure, cardiogenic shock, or acute coronary syndrome resulting from catecholamine-induced acute cardiomyopathy.[3]
- Differential diagnosis of hypertension in pregnancy includes:
  - Gestational hypertension
  - Preeclampsia
  - Eclampsia
  - Pregestational (chronic) hypertension
  - PPGL
- Pregnancy-related hypertension generally presents after 20 weeks gestation; thus, if hypertension is present prior to this, PPGL should be considered.
- Biochemical evaluation
  - If history and clinical findings suggest PPGL, biochemical testing should be performed to evaluate for elevation of catecholamines and/or metanephrines.
  - There is no change in catecholamine metabolism in pregnant individuals when compared to nonpregnant individuals; therefore, the same biochemical testing can be performed regardless of pregnancy status.
  - Various medications can cause false-positive biochemical test results such as methyldopa, labetalol, and tricyclic antidepressants.[7]
- Testing
  - Plasma-free metanephrines or urinary fractionated metanephrines have the highest sensitivity for diagnosing PPGL.[1,2]
  - Metanephrines are recommended preferentially over catecholamines. Plasma or urinary catecholamines within reference range do not exclude the diagnosis of PPGL.[8] Conversely, in almost all patients with PPGL, aside from microscopic tumors, plasma or urinary metanephrines will be elevated (either metanephrine, normetanephrine, or both).[8]
  - Plasma-free metanephrines should be drawn after the patient has been in the supine or seated position for at least 30 minutes.[1]
  - 24-hour urine collection for urinary fractionated metanephrines should be obtained along with a 24-hour urine collection for creatinine in order to ensure a proper sample.
  - When interpreting positive test results, the degree of elevation of urine or plasma metanephrines factors into clinical decision making. Although there are no well-defined guidelines on the degree of elevation which should raise suspicion for PPGL, metanephrines that are two or more times the upper limit of normal range are very suggestive of the diagnosis.[8] In one study, a plasma normetanephrine concentration above 400 ng/L or plasma metanephrine concentration above 236 ng/L raised suspicion for PPGL.[9]
  - Clonidine suppression testing to differentiate between false-positive and true-positive results is contraindicated in pregnancy.[2]
- Tumor localization studies are indicated only after confirmation of biochemical abnormalities indicative of PPGL.
  - Preferred forms of imaging in pregnancy are MRI without gadolinium and abdominal ultrasound.[7]
  - CT scans and functional imaging such as MIBG scintigraphy should not be used in pregnancy.

TREATMENT

- After the diagnosis of PPGL is made and imaging identifies the location of the tumor, treatment consists of α-receptor blockade and subsequent surgery.
  - Use of an α-receptor antagonist helps control downstream effects of catecholamine excess such as hypertension.[9] No guidelines exist for recommended blood pressure targets in pregnant women with catecholamine excess, but caution is needed to avoid dropping blood pressure too low to avoid

compromising uteroplacental circulation. The recommended target blood pressure for treatment of hypertension in pregnancy is 140/90 mmHg, thus it may be reasonable to use this target when treating hypertension secondary to catecholamine excess.[2,10]

- Phenoxybenzamine
  - A noncompetitive α_1- and α_2-receptor antagonist
  - Pregnancy category C
  - Side effects include reflex tachycardia and postoperative hypotension
  - Potential clinical effects last up to a week after discontinuation due to its long half-life of 24 hours[11,12]
  - Crosses the placenta, therefore it is recommended that for the first days of life the newborn be monitored for hypotension and respiratory depression
  - Starting dose is 10 mg twice daily, increasing by 10–20 mg every 2–3 days, with a maximum dose of 1 mg/kg per day[2,11-13]
- Doxazosin
  - A competitive α_1-receptor antagonist
  - Lower risk of reflex tachycardia in comparison to phenoxybenzamine[2]
  - Half-life of approximately 20 hours allows for daily dosing[3,13]
  - Starting dose is 2 mg per day, increasing every 1–2 weeks up to 16 mg daily. Some studies include doses of up to 32 mg daily[2,3]
- Prazosin
  - A selective α_1-receptor antagonist
  - Short half-life of about 2–3 hours so must be dosed 2–3 times per day
  - Starting dose of 1 mg two or three times daily, and a final dose anywhere from 2 to 20 mg daily[3,11-13]
- Other medications
  - Metyrosine
    - Tyrosine hydroxylase inhibitor which decreases synthesis of catecholamines
    - Contraindicated in pregnancy[2,3]
  - β-blockers
    - May be used to control tachycardia

- Should only be initiated after the patient has received α-receptor antagonist therapy for at least 1–2 weeks in order to avoid unopposed α-receptor stimulation and exacerbation of hypertension
- Surgical resection
  - Patients should have at least 10–14 days of α-blockade therapy prior to surgery for PPGL.[3,7]
  - Surgery should be performed before 24 weeks gestation.
  - If the patient is diagnosed with PPGL after 24 weeks gestation, surgical resection can be reserved until the time of delivery if cesarean section is to be performed, or 2–6 weeks after vaginal delivery.[3]
  - A retrospective cohort study and systematic review noted adverse outcomes after surgical resection of PPGL in 8% of pregnancies and that surgical management was not associated with better outcomes. There were no significant adverse outcomes associated with the type of delivery (cesarean section versus vaginal delivery).[6]
  - Preferred surgical procedures are laparoscopic tumor resection for pheochromocytoma and open resection for paraganglioma unless the tumor is located where laparoscopic removal would be feasible.[3,4,7] Therefore, when determining a surgical plan, consideration must be given to gestational age, location of tumor, degree of excess catecholamine secretion control, and surgeon experience.[3]

REFERENCES

1. Lenders JW, Duh QY, Eisenhofer G, et al. Pheochromocytoma and paraganglioma: An Endocrine Society clinical practice guideline. J Clin Endocrinol Metab. 2014;99(6): 1915–1942.
2. Lenders JW, Langton K, Langenhuijsen JF, et al. Pheochromocytoma and pregnancy. Endocrinol Metab Clin N Am. 2019;48: 605–617.

3. Prete A, Paragliola RM, Salvatori R, et al. Management of catecholamine-secreting tumors in pregnancy: A review. Endocr Pract. 2016;22(3): 357–370.

4. Biggar MA, Lennard TW. Systematic review of phaeochromocytoma in pregnancy. Br J Surg. 2013;100: 182–190.

5. Corsello SM, Paragliola RM. Evaluation and management of endocrine hypertension during pregnancy. Endocrinol Metab Clin North Am. 2019;48(4): 829–842.

6. Bancos I, Atkinson E, Eng C, et al. Maternal and fetal outcomes in phaeochromocytoma and pregnancy: A multicentre retrospective cohort study and systematic review of literature. Lancet Diabetes Endocrinol. 2021;9(1): 13–21.

7. Kamoun M, Mnif MF, Charfi N, et al. Adrenal disease during pregnancy: Pathophysiology, diagnosis and management strategies. Am J Med Sci. 2014;347(1): 64–73.

8. Sbardella E, Grossman AB. Pheochromocytoma: An approach to diagnosis. Best Pract Res Clin Endocrinol Metab. 2020;34(2): 101346.

9. Eisenhofer G, Goldstein DS, Walther MM, et al. Biochemical diagnosis of pheochromocytoma: how to distinguish true- from false-positive test results. J Clin Endocrinol Metab. 2003;88(6): 2656–2666.

10. Williams B, Mancia G, Spiering W, et al. 2018 ESC/ESH guidelines for the management of arterial hypertension: The Task Force for the Management of Arterial Hypertension of the European Society of Cardiology and the European Society of Hypertension. J Hypertens. 2018;36(10): 1953–2041.

11. Wing LA, Conaglen JV, Meyer-Rochow GY, et al. Paraganglioma in pregnancy: A case series and review of the literature. J Clin Endocrinol Metab. 2015;100(8): 3202–3209.

12. Eisenhofer G, Rivers G, Rosas AL, et al. Adverse drug reactions in patients with phaeochromocytoma: Incidence, prevention and management. Drug Saf. 2007;30: 1031–1062.

13. Pacak K. Preoperative management of the pheochromocytoma patient. J Clin Endocrinol Metab. 2007 Nov;92(11): 4069–4079.

4c

Primary hyperaldosteronism

VIVEK ALAIGH AND AMANDA FERNANDES

KEY POINTS

- Diagnosis of primary hyperaldosteronism in pregnancy can be challenging as renin and aldosterone levels increase during pregnancy.
- Diagnosis should be based on clinical suspicion in patients with uncontrolled hypertension and hypokalemia.
- Medical management of primary hyperaldosteronism is key to preventing fetal and maternal complications. Many of the agents used in the treatment of nonpregnant individuals with primary hyperaldosteronism cross the placental barrier and can have possible teratogenic effects.
- Surgery can be considered in the second trimester in those with uncontrolled hypertension due to primary hyperaldosteronism.

INTRODUCTION

- Hypertension is present in approximately 10% of pregnancies in the United States. It is associated with several maternal and fetal complications including placental abruption, intrauterine growth restriction, prematurity, and intrauterine death.[1]
- Pregnancy-induced hypertension is defined as a systolic blood pressure >140 mmHg and diastolic blood pressure >90 mmHg.
- Hypertension during pregnancy can be due to:
  - Preexisting hypertension diagnosed before pregnancy or before 20 weeks gestation
  - Gestational hypertension diagnosed at or after 20 weeks gestation
  - Preexisting hypertension with super-imposed gestational hypertension with preeclampsia
  - Unclassifiable hypertension: This category includes hypertension caused by primary hyperaldosteronism, either due to an adrenal adenoma or bilateral adrenal hyperplasia[2]

EPIDEMIOLOGY

- Primary hyperaldosteronism is one of the more common causes of secondary hypertension in the nonpregnant adult population, with a prevalence of 5–10%.[3] Its prevalence in the pregnant population is unknown due to limited data.
- There are over 40 documented case reports of primary hyperaldosteronism in pregnancy, although there is concern of under-diagnosis during pregnancy, possibly due to difficulty in differentiating primary hyperaldosteronism from normal cardiovascular and hormonal changes in pregnancy.

DOI: 10.1201/9781003027577-18

- Most cases of primary hyperaldosteronism were diagnosed prior to conception or during the first trimester.
- Sixty percent of documented cases of primary hyperaldosteronism in pregnancy were caused by a unilateral adrenal adenoma.[4]

PATHOPHYSIOLOGY

- Pregnancy is associated with significant physiologic changes in the cardiovascular system to meet the increasing metabolic demands of the mother and fetus.[5] The renin-angiotensin-aldosterone system (RAAS) plays a key role in meeting these demands. RAAS activation starts around 6–8 weeks into pregnancy and peaks around 28–30 weeks.
- There are several factors that stimulate renin release. The ovaries have been shown to produce prorenin, the precursor protein for renin, which may have a downstream effect on the RAAS.[6] Prorenin levels peak around week 6–8 of gestation.[7] In addition to the ovaries, the placenta also stimulates renin production. It has been estimated that the combination of the extra-renal and renal sources of renin cause the plasma renin activity (PRA) to increase almost 7-fold by the third trimester.[4] Renin levels then drop following delivery.[8]
- Estrogen stimulates hepatic synthesis of angiotensinogen which leads to downstream

activation of the RAAS.[7] Estrogen is also thought to upregulate transcription for angiotensin II receptors, leading to further activation of RAAS.[9]

- Along with estrogen, progesterone levels rise during pregnancy. Progesterone acts as an aldosterone antagonist at the level of the mineralocorticoid receptor and promotes renal excretion of sodium. This natriuresis keeps the RAAS activated and helps prevent hypokalemia.[10]
- The normal physiologic net effect of activation of the RAAS is to increase sodium reabsorption in the proximal convoluted tubule and loop of Henle and increase water retention through vasopressin and aldosterone to cause volume expansion needed for appropriate blood flow to the placenta and fetus.
- Despite the volume expansion with the activation of RAAS during pregnancy, blood pressure is maintained through a number of changes in the cardiovascular system (Figure 4c.1).
  - The rise in plasma volume starting in the first trimester causes an increase in the cardiac output.[5] Output can increase up to 45% in a normal singleton pregnancy by 24 weeks gestation.[5,11]
  - Systemic vascular resistance begins to decrease in the first trimester and reaches its lowest point by the mid-second

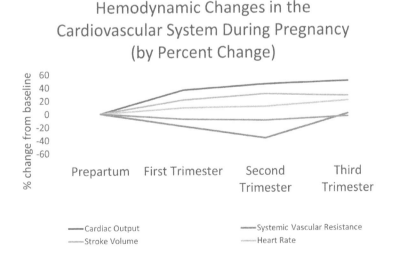

Figure 4c.1 Hemodynamic changes in the cardiovascular system during pregnancy

trimester.[12] Its decrease is approximately 35–45% from baseline, thought to be due to an increase in vascular compliance.[13]

- Several hormones regulate these hemodynamic changes. Relaxin, a hormone created by the corpus luteum which peaks in concentration during the first trimester, has a direct vasodilatory effect and reduces systemic vascular resistance.[14] The degree of vasodilation outmatches the increased cardiac output, typically leading to a decrease in blood pressure during pregnancy.

- Systolic, diastolic, and mean arterial blood pressures all decrease during pregnancy. This reduction occurs at the beginning of pregnancy around 7 weeks gestation and reaches its nadir around the second trimester, as low as 5–10 mmHg from baseline.[15,16] Blood pressure begins to increase around the third trimester and returns to its preconception baseline in the postpartum setting. Heart rate increases by 20–25% during pregnancy, reaching its peak during the third trimester.[5]

DIAGNOSIS

- In nonpregnant individuals with hypertension, an elevated aldosterone/renin ratio (ARR) with suppressed plasma renin activity suggests a diagnosis of primary hyperaldosteronism. During pregnancy, elevated renin and aldosterone can complicate a diagnosis of primary hyperaldosteronism, as the ARR can decrease causing a false negative result.

- Screening should be considered in pregnancy if there is severe hypertension, especially prior to pregnancy or 20th week gestation, with or without hypokalemia.[17]

- A suppressed PRA in the setting of an elevated aldosterone level favors the diagnosis of primary hyperaldosteronism in hypertensive pregnant individuals. However, the antagonistic activity of progesterone during pregnancy can mask primary hyperaldosteronism by lowering aldosterone and normalizing potassium levels. In this situation, primary hyperaldosteronism may not manifest until after delivery, when progesterone levels have decreased.[18]

- Confirmatory testing during pregnancy including saline infusion or oral salt loading is not recommended due to concerns of overexpansion of plasma volume.[4] Similarly, captopril challenge testing is not recommended due to adverse fetal effects of angiotensin-converting enzyme (ACE) inhibitors.[4] In prior cases where saline suppression testing has been done during pregnancy, plasma aldosterone levels did not appropriately suppress.[19–21] An elevated 24-hour urine aldosterone has been used to confirm primary hyperaldosteronism in a few cases.[19]

- If imaging is necessary to evaluate for an adrenal adenoma, the recommended imaging modality is a non-contrast magnetic resonance imaging (MRI) of the adrenal gland.[1,22]

- Adrenal vein sampling to distinguish unilateral from bilateral disease is not recommended during pregnancy and should be deferred until after delivery due to the risk of fetal radiation exposure.[17,22]

TREATMENT

- There are no formal guidelines for management of primary hyperaldosteronism during pregnancy.

- The main goal is treatment of hypertension to prevent fetal and maternal complications. Given that many antihypertensive medications cross the placenta, the treatment for hypertension secondary to primary hyperaldosteronism during pregnancy is similar to treatment of hypertension from other etiologies.

- In pregnancy, α-methyldopa is one of the first-line agents for treatment of hypertension.[22,23] Other medications used for management of hypertension in pregnant patients with primary hyperaldosteronism include hydralazine and calcium channel blockers such as nifedipine.[24–29] ACE inhibitors are contraindicated in pregnancy due to potential toxic effects on the fetus. Recent studies, however, have begun to reevaluate their risk of congenital malformations.

- Mineralocorticoid receptor antagonists such as spironolactone and eplerenone are typically first-line agents in treatment of primary hyperaldosteronism. However, because spironolactone can cross the placenta, there is a concern with its use during pregnancy due to the theoretical risk of feminization of male fetuses based on animal models. Thus, mineralocorticoid receptor antagonists are not recommended for use in pregnancy and should be discontinued approximately one month before conception.[23] In the limited cases of spironolactone use during pregnancy for primary hyperaldosteronism, no feminization or malformations were noted in male infants.[4] There was a single case of sexual ambiguity in a female fetus in the setting of maternal use of spironolactone until the fifth month of pregnancy.[30] No significant data exists regarding the use of eplerenone during pregnancy.[19]

- Though diuretics are not typically used for hypertension in pregnancy, the potassium-sparing diuretic, amiloride, has been used with good effect in pregnancy complicated by primary hyperaldosteronism.[31,32]
- If an aldosterone-producing adrenal adenoma is diagnosed prior to pregnancy, surgical resection is recommended. If diagnosed during pregnancy, adrenalectomy can be considered during the second trimester for those with refractory hypertension.[33-38]

REFERENCES

1. Abdelmannan D, Aron DC. Adrenal disorders in pregnancy. *Endocrinol Metab Clin North Am*. Dec 2011;40(4):779–94.
2. Mustafa R, Ahmed S, Gupta A, Venuto R. A comprehensive review of hypertension in pregnancy. *J Pregnancy*. 2012;2012:105918.
3. Funder JW, Carey RM, Mantero F, et al. The management of primary aldosteronism: Case detection, diagnosis, and treatment: An Endocrine Society Clinical Practice guideline. *J Clin Endocrinol Metab*. 2016;101(5):1889–916.
4. Morton A. Primary aldosteronism and pregnancy. *Pregnancy Hypertens*. 2015;5(4):259–62.
5. Sanghavi M, Rutherford JD. Cardiovascular physiology of pregnancy. *Circulation*. 2014;130(12):1003–8.
6. Sealey JE, McCord D, Taufield PA, et al. Plasma prorenin in first-trimester pregnancy: Relationship to changes in human chorionic gonadotropin. *Am J Obstet Gynecol*. 1985;153(5):514–19.
7. Lumbers ER, Pringle KG. Roles of the circulating renin-angiotensin-aldosterone system in human pregnancy. *Am J Physiol Regul Integr Comp Physiol*. 2014;306(2):R91–101.
8. Hsueh WA, Luetscher JA, Carlson EJ, Grislis G, Fraze E, McHargue A. Changes in active and inactive renin throughout pregnancy. *J Clin Endocrinol Metab*. 1982;54(5):1010–16.
9. Sampson AK, Hilliard LM, Moritz KM, et al. The arterial depressor response to chronic low-dose angiotensin II infusion in female rats is estrogen dependent. *Am J Physiol Regul Integr Comp Physiol*. 2012;302(1):R159–65.
10. Oelkers W. Antimineralocorticoid activity of a novel oral contraceptive containing drospirenone, a unique progestogen resembling natural progesterone. *Eur J Contracept Reprod Health Care*. 2002;7(suppl 3):19–26.
11. Hunter S, Robson SC. Adaptation of the maternal heart in pregnancy. *Br Heart J*. 1992;68(6):540–43.
12. Mahendru AA, Everett TR, Wilkinson IB, Lees CC, McEniery CM. A longitudinal study of maternal cardiovascular function from preconception to the postpartum period. *J Hypertens*. 2014;32(4):849–856.
13. Clapp JF, Capeless E. Cardiovascular function before, during, and after the first and subsequent pregnancies. *Am J Cardiol*. 1997;80(11):1469–73.
14. Fisher C, MacLean M, Morecroft I, et al. Is the pregnancy hormone relaxin also a vasodilator peptide secreted by the heart? *Circulation*. 2002;106(3):292–95.
15. Grindheim G, Estensen ME, Langesaeter E, Rosseland LA, Toska K. Changes in blood pressure during healthy pregnancy: A longitudinal cohort study. *J Hypertens*. 2012;30(2):342–50.
16. Ouzounian JG, Elkayam U. Physiologic changes during normal pregnancy and delivery. *Cardiol Clin*. 2012;30(3):317–29.
17. Riester A, Reincke M. Progress in primary aldosteronism: Mineralocorticoid receptor antagonists and management of

primary aldosteronism in pregnancy. *Eur J Endocrinol*. 2015;172(1):R23–30.

18. Ronconi V, Turchi F, Zennaro MC, Boscaro M, Giacchetti G. Progesterone increase counteracts aldosterone action in a pregnant woman with primary aldosteronism. *Clin Endocrinol (Oxf)*. 2011;74(2):278–79.

19. Cabassi A, Rocco R, Berretta R, Regolisti G, Bacchi-Modena A. Eplerenone use in primary aldosteronism during pregnancy. *Hypertension*. 2012;59(2):e18–e19.

20. Neerhof MG, Shlossman PA, Poll DS, Ludomirsky A, Weiner S. Idiopathic aldosteronism in pregnancy. *Obstet Gynecol*. 1991;78(3 Pt 2):489–91.

21. Shalhav AL, Landman J, Afane J, Levi R, Clayman RV. Laparoscopic adrenalectomy for primary hyperaldosteronism during pregnancy. *J Laparoendosc Adv Surg Tech A*. 2000;10(3):169–71.

22. Young WF. Diagnosis and treatment of primary aldosteronism: Practical clinical perspectives. *J Intern Med*. 2019;285(2):126–48.

23. Landau E, Amar L. Primary aldosteronism and pregnancy. *Ann Endocrinol (Paris)*. 2016;77(2):148–60.

24. Kosaka K, Onoda N, Ishikawa T, et al. Laparoscopic adrenalectomy on a patient with primary aldosteronism during pregnancy. *Endocr J*. 2006;53(4):461–66.

25. Lotgering FK, Derkx FM, Wallenburg HC. Primary hyperaldosteronism in pregnancy. *Am J Obstet Gynecol*. 1986;155(5):986–88.

26. Lu W, Zheng F, Li H, Ruan L. Primary aldosteronism and pregnancy: A case report. *Aust N Z J Obstet Gynaecol*. 2009;49(5):558.

27. Fujiyama S, Mori Y, Matsubara H, et al. Primary aldosteronism with aldosterone-producing adrenal adenoma in a pregnant woman. *Intern Med*. 1999;38(1):36–39.

28. Schlienger JL, Duval J, Langer B, Jaeck D, Schlaeder G. Conn's adenoma in pregnancy. *Presse Med*. 1990;19(39):1810.

29. Wang W, Long W, Li G, Yang H. Primary aldosteronism in pregnancy: Review of cases. *Chin Med J (Engl)*. 1999;112(6):574–75.

30. Shah A. Ambiguous genitalia in a newborn with spironolactone exposure (abstract). *Presented at the 93rd Annual Meeting of the Endocrine Society*, Boston, MA. 2017;4:227.

31. Krysiak R, Samborek M, Stojko R. Primary aldosteronism in pregnancy. *Acta Clin Belg*. 2012;67(2):130–34.

32. Al-Ali NA, El-Sandabesee D, Steel SA, Roland JM. Conn's syndrome in pregnancy successfully treated with amiloride. *J Obstet Gynaecol*. 2007;27(7):730–31.

33. Aboud E, De Swiet M, Gordon H. Primary aldosteronism in pregnancy–should it be treated surgically? *Ir J Med Sci*. 1995;164(4):279–80.

34. Baron F, Sprauve ME, Huddleston JF, Fisher AJ. Diagnosis and surgical treatment of primary aldosteronism in pregnancy: A case report. *Obstet Gynecol*. 1995;86(4 Pt 2):644–45.

35. Gordon RD, Fishman LM, Liddle GW. Plasma renin activity and aldosterone secretion in a pregnant woman with primary aldosteronism. *J Clin Endocrinol Metab*. 1967;27(3):385–88.

36. Nursal TZ, Caliskan K, Ertorer E, Parlakgumus A, Moray G. Laparoscopic treatment of primary hyperaldosteronism in a pregnant patient. *Can J Surg*. 2009;52(5):E188–90.

37. Shigematsu K, Nishida N, Sakai H, et al. Primary aldosteronism with aldosterone-producing adenoma consisting of pure zona glomerulosa-type cells in a pregnant woman. *Endocr Pathol*. 2009;20(1):66–72.

38. Solomon CG, Thiet M, Moore F, Seely EW. Primary hyperaldosteronism in pregnancy. A case report. *J Reprod Med. Apr* 1996;41(4):255–58.

Cushing's syndrome

ELA BANERJEE AND VICKY CHENG

KEY POINTS

- Pregnancy is rare in Cushing's syndrome due to anovulatory infertility induced by excess cortisol.
- Adrenal adenoma is the most common cause of Cushing's syndrome in pregnant patients.
- Pregnancy leads to physiologic hypercortisolism, making the diagnosis of Cushing's syndrome challenging.
- Cushing's syndrome in pregnancy increases maternal risk of gestational diabetes mellitus, gestational hypertension, and preeclampsia. It also increases risk of fetal morbidity and mortality.
- There is no definitive diagnostic algorithm for Cushing's syndrome in pregnancy and the usual tests to evaluate for hypercortisolism are confounded by physiologic hypercortisolism of pregnancy. One proposed criterion includes urinary free cortisol >3-fold the upper limit of normal (ULN) and late-night salivary cortisol >3-fold ULN in patients presenting with symptoms suggestive of Cushing's syndrome.
- Treatment of Cushing's syndrome in pregnancy involves surgical or medical therapy. Surgery leads to more successful outcomes than medical therapy alone. Even in treated cases, however, complications such as preeclampsia and premature delivery are common.

EPIDEMIOLOGY

- Cushing's syndrome has an incidence of 2–25 cases per million per year in the general population.[1]
- Causes of Cushing's syndrome in the nonpregnant population:
  - Adrenocorticotropic hormone (ACTH)-secreting pituitary adenoma (70%)
    - Also known as Cushing's disease[1,2]
    - Incidence of 1.2–2.4 cases per million per year
    - Prevalence of 1.2–5.6% of all pituitary tumors
    - Higher female prevalence with a 3–4:1 ratio. For women, the incidence peaks at ages 30–40s
  - Adrenal adenoma (15%)[2,3]
  - Other causes including ectopic ACTH secretion, pheochromocytoma, and Carney complex (15%)
- Causes of Cushing's syndrome in pregnancy[4]:
  - Adrenal adenoma (60%)
  - ACTH-secreting pituitary adenoma (33%)
  - Ectopic ACTH secretion (7%)
  - Less common causes include pheochromocytoma and adrenal hyperplasia

DOI: 10.1201/9781003027577-19

- Pregnancy is uncommon in women with untreated Cushing's syndrome. Cushing's syndrome typically results in anovulatory infertility as uncontrolled hypercortisolism inhibits normal development of ovarian follicles and ovulation. Nevertheless, over 260 cases of Cushing's syndrome in pregnancy have been reported.
- While Cushing's disease is the most common etiology of excess cortisol in the general population, adrenal adenoma is the most common cause in pregnancy.
- The increased incidence of adrenal hypercortisolism leading to Cushing's syndrome during pregnancy is not well-understood.[5] It has been suggested that Cushing's disease leads to hypersecretion of both cortisol and adrenal androgens. This hyperandrogenic state results in amenorrhea in over 70% of cases of Cushing's disease. However, in those with adrenal Cushing's syndrome with typically isolated hypercortisolism, ovulation may be less frequently suppressed.[2-5]
- Patients with ectopic ACTH secretion have severe hypercortisolism and amenorrhea making pregnancy even less prevalent.
- Pregnancies in women with Cushing's syndrome are associated with high rates of maternal complications and fetal morbidity with at least 20% fetal mortality.[5]
- A systematic review compared characteristics of active versus cured Cushing's syndrome in pregnant women.[1] Results of this study are summarized in Table 4d.1.

PATHOPHYSIOLOGY

- Normal pregnancy consists of a state of physiologic hypercortisolism due to activation of the maternal hypothalamic-pituitary-adrenal (HPA) axis.[4,6] However, the physiologic hypercortisolism of pregnancy does not lead to clinical manifestations of Cushing's syndrome such as large violaceous abdominal striae, proximal muscle weakness, cutaneous atrophy, osteoporosis, or heart failure.[4]
- Corticotropin-releasing hormone (CRH) physiology
  - CRH is normally synthesized in the hypothalamus. The placenta also synthesizes and releases biologically active CRH. There is an exponential rise in CRH secretion from the placenta by 1000-fold beginning at 8 weeks gestation. This production peaks at 40 weeks, preceding onset of labor.[5-7]
  - The CRH level later normalizes to non-pregnant levels within 24 hours of delivery. Placental CRH assists with development and maturation of the fetal HPA axis and fetal adrenal glands resulting in fetal adrenal steroidogenesis.[4-7] The placental CRH acts on the maternal HPA axis as well and triggers increased maternal cortisol production.
- ACTH physiology
  - In addition to maternal CRH-stimulated pituitary release of ACTH, there is also direct release of ACTH from the placenta.

Table 4d.1 Summary of data from Caimari et al. reviewing causes of hypercortisolism and frequency of complications associated with Cushing's in pregnancy

	Active CS	Cured CS	p-Value
Number of patients (%)	214 (81.4%)	49 (18.6%)	
Age at diagnosis	28.9 ± 5.2 years	30.4 ± 5.6 years	$p = 0.075$
Hypercortisolism etiology	Adrenal adenoma (44.1%)	Pituitary Cushing's disease (73%)	$p < 0.001$
Gestational age at delivery	34 weeks	39 weeks	$p < 0.001$
Delivery via C-section	51.7%	21.9%	$p = 0.003$
Gestational diabetes	36.9%	2.3%	$p = 0.003$
Gestational hypertension	40.5%	2.3%	$p < 0.001$
Preeclampsia	26.3%	2.3%	$p = 0.001$
Fetal loss	23.6%	8.5%	$p = 0.021$
Fetal morbidity	33.3%	4.9%	$p < 0.001$
Preterm birth	65.8%	2.56%	$p < 0.001$

Furthermore, there is blunting of maternal normal feedback control on ACTH that results in exponential increase in ACTH levels.[5] ACTH levels peak during labor and delivery, almost 3-fold above those in the first trimester. Nevertheless, the diurnal pattern of plasma ACTH secretion is preserved during normal pregnancy.

- Placental CRH and ACTH lead to maternal adrenal gland hypertrophy during pregnancy and increased production of cortisol. Elevated levels of cortisol help activate the cascade of intracellular signaling which results in induction of labor. CRH receptors have been found on the myometrial smooth muscles in the uterus and CRH may also contribute to onset of labor.[7]
- Hypercortisolism in pregnancy
  - Gestational Cushing's syndrome results in an uncontrolled and unregulated rise in maternal cortisol production, leading to increased risk of gestational diabetes mellitus (GDM), gestational hypertension, and preeclampsia. Other complications of supraphysiologic hypercortisolism include poor wound healing, osteoporosis, fractures, psychiatric manifestations, maternal cardiac failure, and death.[5]
  - GDM
    - Hypercortisolism impairs fasting and postprandial glucose values.
    - Cortisol increases gluconeogenesis by upregulating gluconeogenic enzymes.
    - Cortisol induces selective insulin resistance which prevents the inhibitory effect of insulin on hepatic glucose output.
    - Cortisol also increases the rate of muscle breakdown, leading to loss of muscle mass, decreased muscle insulin responsiveness, and impaired glucose uptake.[8]
    - 11ß-hydroxysteroid dehydrogenase (11ß-HSD) type 1 is an enzyme located in liver and adipose tissue. It converts biologically inactive cortisone to cortisol, therefore its increased activity in the setting of hypercortisolism intensifies insulin resistance.[8]
  - Gestational hypertension
    - 11ß-HSD type 2 converts cortisol to cortisone and is highly expressed by the placenta and mineralocorticoid receptor (MR) target tissues like the renal cortex. By inactivating cortisol, 11ß-HSD2 prevents binding of cortisol to MR.[4,5,8–10]
    - In Cushing's syndrome, high cortisol concentrations overwhelm 11ß-HSD2, leading to MR activation and causing increased renal tubular sodium reabsorption and increased intravascular expansion.
    - Cortisol also directly acts on angiotensin II, decreases nitric oxide activity, promotes endothelial damage, and increases vascular permeability, all of which worsen hypertension.[10]
  - Preeclampsia
    - Cortisol is detectable in the placenta of up to 80% of preeclampsia-associated pregnancies while most normotensive pregnancies have absence of placental cortisol.[11]
    - At the placental level, the action of 11ß-HSD2 protects the fetus from high levels of maternal cortisol. Gestational Cushing's syndrome results in both over-saturation and dysregulation of placental 11ß-HSD2 and therefore high levels of placental cortisol, leading to low fetal birth weight and preeclampsia.[8,11]
- Osteoporosis
  - Cortisol excess inhibits bone formation and increases bone resorption. It also impairs intestinal absorption of calcium and secretion of growth hormone and gonadotropins that affect bone metabolism, resulting in bone loss and osteoporotic fractures.[12]

DIAGNOSIS

- Biochemical diagnosis of Cushing's syndrome is difficult to establish due to the physiologic hypercortisolism of pregnancy resulting in elevation of plasma cortisol, cortisol-binding globulin (CBG), urinary free cortisol (UFC), and late-night salivary cortisol.[1,4–6,13]
- Clinical findings
  - Pregnant patients with Cushing's syndrome develop weight gain, hypertension,

bruising, and hirsutism, yet Cushing's syndrome is typically not detected until 12–26 weeks gestation, partially because the physical changes can be attributed to the pregnant state as well.

- Symptoms such as muscle weakness, large violaceous striae in regions outside the abdomen, and osteoporosis are suggestive of Cushing's syndrome instead of normal pregnancy.[3]
- Free cortisol
  - In normal pregnancy, the serum free cortisol increases by approximately 1.6-fold by the 11th week of pregnancy and up to 2- to 3-fold as pregnancy progresses.
  - UFC increases up to 3-fold during the second and third trimesters of pregnancy.
  - Late-night salivary cortisol, which is also a measure of free cortisol, increases by 2- to 3-fold.
- CBG:
  - Increased placental production of estradiol stimulates hepatic production of CBG, reaching its highest level at the end of pregnancy and consequently increasing circulating levels of bound cortisol. This protects the mother from the harmful effects of physiologic hypercortisolism.
  - Increased CBG results in elevated total cortisol levels, thus the 1 mg dexamethasone suppression test for screening of Cushing's syndrome becomes unreliable, with high rates of false-positives in pregnant patients as the morning plasma or serum cortisol includes a measurement of total, rather than free, cortisol.[5]
- Postpartum, levels of plasma CRH, ACTH, and cortisol fall rapidly to nonpregnant ranges consistent with their biological half-lives.[5]
- Even though adrenal adenoma is the primary cause of Cushing's syndrome during pregnancy, a suppressed ACTH level is typically not seen in these patients due to the physiologic hypercortisolism state of pregnancy as noted above.[4,5]
- Diagnostic testing options
  - Establishing excess cortisol
    - There is no screening or diagnostic algorithm for the diagnosis of Cushing's syndrome during pregnancy.
    - The Endocrine Society suggests that a combination of UFC levels >3 times ULN and midnight salivary cortisol levels >3 times ULN during the second and third trimesters of pregnancy can be used to screen for Cushing's syndrome in pregnancy.
    - Cortisol secretion maintains a pulsatile and circadian rhythm during normal pregnancy, therefore loss of this circadian pulsatility is indicative of Cushing's syndrome as well.[5,13]
  - Establishing cause
    - Once Cushing's syndrome is confirmed, ACTH should be measured to determine ACTH-dependent versus ACTH-independent etiology.
    - As most pregnant patients with Cushing's syndrome have a normal or elevated ACTH regardless of etiology, a low-normal ACTH can indicate ACTH-independent disease, and should prompt imaging of the adrenal glands.
    - If ACTH is not suppressed, 8 mg dexamethasone suppression testing can distinguish between excess pituitary and ectopic ACTH production. Although CRH stimulation testing may be done in nonpregnant patients, CRH is an FDA category C medication and its use in pregnancy should be limited.[5,13]
- Inferior petrosal sinus sampling (IPSS)
  - This procedure may be necessary in some cases with discordant biochemical and/or imaging findings to help diagnose Cushing's disease as a cause of Cushing's syndrome.
  - It should only be considered in pregnancy after all noninvasive assessments have been completed and should only be attempted at experienced centers.
  - There is concern regarding the use of radiation during this testing which limits its application in pregnancy.[13]
- Imaging
  - Imaging of the adrenal glands helps to identify adrenal Cushing's syndrome. Ultrasound imaging has been shown to be safe and effective; however, it is less sensitive when the tumor size is small. MRI and CT scans are also available imaging modalities; however, MRI

is preferred in pregnant women after 32 weeks gestation.

– Imaging of the pituitary gland with MRI assists with diagnosis of Cushing's disease. Nevertheless, there are several caveats to imaging the pituitary gland during pregnancy. The pituitary gland normally increases in size by up to 2-fold over the course of pregnancy. Thus, if nonpregnant size criteria are used to assess pituitary lesions in a pregnant woman, physiologic changes may be incorrectly labeled as pituitary adenomas. Additionally, MRI is not routinely performed during the first trimester due to potential concerns for teratogenic effects during organogenesis but is considered safe after 32 weeks gestation. Gadolinium use is not advised in pregnancy as it is an FDA category C drug, therefore resulting in decreased sensitivity of the imaging as well. As a result, the risks versus benefits must be considered when performing MRI in pregnant patients between 12 and 32 weeks gestation.[5,13]

TREATMENT

- Although the adverse effects of untreated Cushing's syndrome on maternal and fetal outcomes may be controlled by decreasing UFC to the ULN of pregnancy range, this concept is not well studied.[5]
- There is no consensus regarding treatment for Cushing's syndrome in pregnancy, however surgery can be considered during second trimester if an adrenal or pituitary adenoma has been identified.[9]
- Surgical options include unilateral versus bilateral adrenalectomy in patients with adrenal Cushing's syndrome and transsphenoidal surgery (TSS) in those with Cushing's disease.[5] One study which evaluated pregnant women with Cushing's syndrome who underwent treatment with TSS, adrenalectomy, external pituitary radiation, or medical therapy noted progression to eclampsia and premature delivery in a significant number of patients despite successful treatment and disease remission.[13]
- Early administration of hydrocortisone perioperatively is recommended to decrease the risk of adrenal crisis.[9]

Table 4d.2 Medical treatment options for Cushing's syndrome in pregnant patients

Medication	Mechanism of action	Comments
Metyrapone Dose: 0.5–3 g/day	11ß-hydroxylase inhibitor	• Generally well-tolerated • Used most often with minimal adverse effects on maternal hepatic function or fetal development[5] • Concern for exacerbation of hypertension and progression to preeclampsia limits its use[5] • One known case of adrenal insufficiency due to its use[3] • Crosses the placenta in animal studies but no neonatal abnormalities have been reported in humans[1,4]
Ketoconazole Dose: 0.6–1.0 g/day	11ß-hydroxylase and 17,20-lyase inhibitor	• Used successfully for treatment of Cushing's syndrome; however, FDA category C drug due to its ability to cross the placenta in animal studies resulting in teratogenicity and abortion • Antiandrogenic effects inhibit aromatase activity • Recommended for patients needing emergent medical therapy who cannot tolerate metyrapone[5]
Cabergoline Dose: 2.0–3.5 mg/wk	Dopamine agonist	• Decreases CRH production in Cushing's disease[6] • One case report of its use prior to 2016[3]

- Medical therapy may be initiated during second or third trimesters for treatment of Cushing's syndrome, although considered second-line following surgery due to side effects (Table 4d.2).[1,4]
- Contraindicated, ineffective, or under-studied medical treatments
  - Cyproheptadine reduced ACTH secretion and was safely used in three cases; however, it was not effective.[5]
  - Aminoglutethimide inhibits several steps along the steroid biosynthesis pathway.[6] It should be avoided due to fetal masculinization and teratogenic effects.[3,5]
  - Mitotane is an adrenolytic agent that directly suppresses the adrenal cortex and alters peripheral metabolism of steroids. Its use is contraindicated in pregnancy due to teratogenic effects.[1,4,5]
  - Radiotherapy is contraindicated during pregnancy due to delayed results and teratogenic effects.[1,4]
  - Pasireotide, a somatostatin analog, has a lack of published data and studies in pregnancy.[14]

REFERENCES

1. Caimari F, Valassi E, Garbayo P, et al. Cushing's Syndrome and Pregnancy Outcomes: A Systematic Review of Published Cases, Endocrine. 2017;55: 555–563.
2. Barbot M, et al. Cushing's Syndrome: Overview of Clinical Presentation, Diagnostic Tools and Complications, Best Practice & Research Clinical Endocrinology & Metabolism. 2020;34: 101380.
3. Bronstein MD, Machado MC, Fragoso MCBV, Management of Pregnant Patients with Cushing's Syndrome, European Journal of Endocrinology. 2015;173: R85–R91.
4. Machado MC, Fragoso MC, Bronstein MD. Pregnancy in Patients with Cushing's Syndrome, Endocrinology and Metabolism Clinics of North America. 2018;47: 441–449.
5. Lindsay JR, Nieman LK. The Hypothalamic-Pituitary-Adrenal Axis in Pregnancy: Challenges in Disease Detection and Treatment, Endocrine Reviews. 2005;26(6): 775–799.
6. Buescher MA, McClamrock HD, Adashi EY. Cushing Syndrome in Pregnancy, Obstetrics and Gynecology. 1992;79(1): 130–137.
7. Grammatopoulos DK. Placental Corticotrophin-Releasing Hormone and Its Receptors in Human Pregnancy and Labour: Still a Scientific Enigma, Journal of Neuroendocrinology. 2018;20: 432–438.
8. Barbot M, Ceccato F, Scaroni C. Diabetes Mellitus Secondary to Cushing's Disease, Front Endocrinol (Lausanne). 2018;9:284.
9. Mellor A, Harvey RD, Pobereskin LH, Sneyd JR. Cushing's Disease Treated by Transsphenoidal Selective Adenomectomy in Mid-Pregnancy, British Journal of Anaesthesia. 1998;80(6): 850–852.
10. Cicala MV, Mantero F. Hypertension in Cushing's Syndrome: From Pathogenesis to Treatment, Neuroendocrinology. 2010;92(1): 44–49.
11. Hogg K, Blair JD, McFadden DE, von Dadelszen P, Robinson WP. Early Onset Pre-Eclampsia Is Associated with Altered DNA Methylation of Cortisol-Signaling and Steroidogenic Genes in the Placenta, PLoS One. 2013;8(5): e62969.
12. Holgado-Galicia MV, Magno JD, Acelajado-Valdenor C, Isip-Tan IT, Lim-Abraham MA. Cushing's Syndrome in Pregnancy, BMJ Case Reports. 2011;2011: bcr0120113720.
13. Lindsay JR, Jonklaas J, Oldfield EH, Nieman LK. Cushing's Syndrome during Pregnancy: Personal Experience and Review of the Literature, Journal of Clinical Endocrinology & Metabolism. 2005; 90(5); 3077–3083.
14. Brue T, Amodru V, Castinetti F. Management of Cushing's Syndrome during Pregnancy: Solved and Unsolved Questions, European Journal of Endocrinology. 2018;178(6): R259–R266.

4e

Adrenocortical carcinoma

DUSHYANTHY ARASARATNAM, NADIA BARGHOUTHI,
AND VLADIMER BAKHUTASHVILI

KEY POINTS

- Adrenocortical carcinomas (ACCs) are rarely diagnosed in pregnancy, with most data in this population derived from case reports.
- Adrenocortical carcinomas have a poor prognosis in both pregnant and nonpregnant patients.
- Diagnosis should include biochemical testing for hypercortisolism, hyperandrogenism, hyperaldosteronism, and excess metanephrine and catecholamine production.

- Surgical resection with postoperative mitotane therapy following delivery is currently considered best practice for treatment of ACC in pregnancy.
- Since most of these tumors produce excess cortisol, hydrocortisone should be initiated peri-operatively to prevent post-operative adrenal insufficiency following surgical resection.

EPIDEMIOLOGY

- Adrenal tumors are common and affect 3–10% of the general population, with the majority consisting of benign adenomas without significant hormone production. In contrast, adrenocortical carcinoma (ACC) is a notably rare disease with incidence around 1–2 cases per million per year.[1]
- ACC has a bimodal age distribution with an initial peak in childhood before the age of five and a subsequent rise during the fourth and fifth decades of life.[2,3] There is increased incidence in women with an earlier median age of discovery, approximately 43 years of age versus 48, when compared to men.[2,4]
- In pregnancy, there is a relative increase in incidence of ACC suggesting elevated estrogen as a risk factor. Contraceptive use in women

and smoking in men has also been found to increase risk.[1,5]

- Prognosis of ACC has more recently been categorized according to the European Network for the Study of Adrenal Tumors (ENSAT) staging system, with tumors limited to 5 cm in size without extra adrenal extension (ENSAT 1) having a survival of 80% at 10 years and tumors larger than 5 cm without extra adrenal involvement (ENSAT 2) having a survival of 60%. Extension to adjacent tissues or lymph nodes (ENSAT 3) drops survival to 40% and distant metastases (ENSAT 4) decrease the survival to 10% at 10 years.[1,4]
- One French case series including 12 pregnant patients (matched with nonpregnant patients) found the survival rate of ACC diagnosed during pregnancy was 50% at 1 year, 28% at 3 years, and 13% at 5 and 8 years with the

DOI: 10.1201/9781003027577-20

diagnosis during pregnancy or in the immediate postpartum period being an independent predictor of poor prognosis.[4]

- Reported complications of ACC in pregnancy include[4]:
  - Premature birth
  - Intrauterine growth restriction
  - Intrauterine fetal demise
  - Maternal postpartum hemorrhage
  - Hypertension
  - Diabetes mellitus
  - Eclampsia
  - Hemolysis, elevated liver enzymes, low platelet count (HELLP) syndrome

PATHOPHYSIOLOGY

- Although germline TP53 mutations are the underlying genetic cause of ACC in up to 80% of children, these mutations occur in only 3–7% of adults with ACC.[1] Other hereditary cancer syndromes associated with ACC include[1,3]:
  - Beckwith-Wiedemann syndrome
  - Multiple endocrine neoplasia (MEN) type 1
  - Familial adenomatous polyposis
  - Neurofibromatosis type 1
  - Werner syndrome
- All ACCs stem from monoclonal cell populations and most commonly involve IGF-2 overexpression and constitutive activation of the Wnt/beta-catenin pathway among other genetic abnormalities.[1,2]
- About 50–60% of ACCs secrete excess hormones, with cortisol and androgens being the most commonly produced.[2,3]

DIAGNOSIS

- The diagnosis of ACC during pregnancy remains extremely rare, with most of the available literature coming from case reports. The scarcity of available literature on ACC in pregnancy is in part due to the overall rarity of ACC, the lower fertility of women with hormone-secreting tumors, as well as the challenges in distinguishing the signs and symptoms of the disease from the pregnant state.[6,7]
- In nonpregnant patients, 40–60% of patients present with signs of hormone excess.[1] In pregnancy, available literature suggests that

almost all tumors present with features of hypercortisolism and/or hyperandrogenism.[8] Typically, glucocorticoid excess comprises 50–80% of hormone-secreting ACCs, adrenal androgens 40–60%, and autonomous aldosterone production is rare, making up only 2–7% of cases. Concurrent cortisol and androgen secretion are evident in half of all ACCs with hormone production.[6] In pregnancy, this proportion appears to be even greater, with one study documenting 12 cases of ACC of which all patients demonstrated hypercortisolism and 75% had cosecretion of androgens.[8]

- The approach to patients suspected of having ACC includes biochemical and radiologic assessment. Biochemical evaluation allows for determination of the tumor biology and diagnosis, prognostication (as glucocorticoid secreting tumors have been associated with more aggressive disease), guidance for hormone replacement requirements following resection, and establishment of potential tumor markers for surveillance.[6] Biochemical assessment requires evaluation of glucocorticoids, mineralocorticoids, androgens, and catecholamines. Pregnancy poses a unique challenge, as the fetal-placental unit alters the maternal hormonal metabolism and feedback mechanisms.

Laboratory evaluation

- Assessment of a mass suspicious for ACC usually begins with cortisol levels following a 1 mg dexamethasone suppression test (DST) and basal adrenocorticotropic hormone (ACTH) levels to establish ACTH independence.[6]
  - This is confirmed with midnight salivary cortisol or 24-hour urine free cortisol (UFC). The evaluation of these levels in pregnancy is complex and the usual diagnostic parameters do not apply.
  - ACTH levels in pregnancy have been reported as normal or elevated in all patients with Cushing's syndrome, including those with ACTH-independent (adrenal) disease.[9] Half of pregnant patients with adrenal Cushing's syndrome fail to suppress ACTH.[10]
  - Pregnancy is a state of hypercortisolism, with a rise in plasma cortisol levels 2- to

3-fold above the normal range. Physiologic elevations in total and free serum cortisol, UFC, and ACTH are seen.[9] Despite this, diurnal variation is preserved.[11]

- Diagnosis of cortisol excess in pregnancy is made using 24-hour UFC or midnight salivary or plasma cortisol levels. As the hypothalamic-pituitary-adrenal (HPA) axis loses sensitivity to the effects of dexamethasone, more than 80% of DSTs in normal pregnancies produce false-positive results, an effect that lasts up to 5 weeks postpartum.[2,5] In a case series of Cushing's syndrome in pregnancy including data from 136 pregnancies in 122 women, a mean 8-fold increase in UFC levels and loss of diurnal variation were seen. The Endocrine Society recommends UFC >3 times the upper limit of normal in second or third trimester be used for the diagnosis of hypercortisolism in pregnancy and recommends against the use of the DST. Identifying a lack of diurnal variation is helpful. Unfortunately, no normative data is available for plasma cortisol in this setting and the use of salivary cortisol in pregnancy has not been validated.[2,9]
- Additional adrenocortical steroid hormone precursors such as 17-hydroxyprogesterone, androstenedione, and 11-deoxycortisol are helpful in assessing an adrenal mass suspicious for ACC.[6] Steroid hormone synthesis in ACCs is relatively inefficient compared to the normal adrenal cortex, therefore urine steroid profiling can reveal increased precursors and metabolites, even in hormonally nonfunctional ACCs.[1]
- Individual steroid metabolite profiles can also be used to monitor for recurrence, progression, and treatment response.[6] Plasma 17-hydroxysteroids, corticosterone, deoxycortisol, and cortisone can all rise during pregnancy, mirroring the 2- to 3-fold rise of cortisol.[9] This makes the use of these steroid precursors challenging, as normative data ranges for pregnancy have not been established.
- DHEA-S and testosterone should be measured in every patient suspected of having ACC.[1] Androgens commonly rise during pregnancy, although reference ranges have not been elucidated for pregnancy.[9] Adrenocortical tumors have been shown to secrete androgens in

response to hCG. Testosterone, dihydrotestosterone, and dehydroepiandrosterone have been shown to increase in response to hCG.[12]
- Screening for hyperaldosteronism requires analysis of plasma renin activity (PRA) and plasma aldosterone concentration (PAC).[1] In nonpregnant individuals, an aldosterone/renin ratio >20 and PAC >10 ng/dL with a concomitantly suppressed renin are accepted as a positive screen.[2] In pregnancy, PRA increases 3- to 7-fold and PAC 5- to 20-fold during gestation. Despite the significant increase in aldosterone concentration, its secretion continues to be governed by normal physiologic stimuli such as posture.[9] Some of the clinical features of hyperaldosteronism can be masked by progesterone which has anti-mineralocorticoid effects.[2]
- Plasma metanephrines should be evaluated in any indeterminate adrenal mass to rule out pheochromocytoma, as it cannot be differentiated from ACC on cross-sectional imaging alone.[6] Catecholamine levels are not altered in pregnancy, allowing a laboratory diagnosis of pheochromocytoma that is similar to the nonpregnant state.[2]

Imaging

- ACCs are typically large, measuring >4 cm, and heterogeneous with central necrosis and hemorrhage.[1] To limit fetal radiation exposure, ultrasound and MRI are used to screen for and characterize adrenal lesions. Gadolinium is an FDA category C drug, and therefore not used in the characterization of these masses.
- On MRI, ACCs demonstrate heterogeneous signal dropout and are isointense or hypointense in comparison to the liver parenchyma on T1-weighted images and hyperintense on T2-weighted images. Postcontrast images demonstrate predominantly irregular peripheral enhancement with central nonenhancing areas secondary to hemorrhage or necrosis. High signal intensity on T1-weighted images is due to internal hemorrhage whereas high signal intensity on T2-weighted images typically represents areas of necrosis.
- Calcifications may be seen in up to 30% of ACCs; however, they can also be seen with other pathology and are not a distinguishing feature. On chemical-shift MRI, intracellular

lipid can cause regions of signal loss on out-of-phase images relative to in-phase images. Direct invasion of local organs may be better demonstrated on MRI due to its multiplanar capability.[1]

TREATMENT

- There is limited data regarding treatment options for ACC diagnosed during pregnancy.
- Pregnancy is suspected to lead to an increased likelihood of relapse and tumor growth.[1]
- Poor fetal outcomes have been reported for women diagnosed with advanced disease during pregnancy or in the immediate postpartum period with intrauterine growth restriction, premature birth, and intrauterine death.
- ACC-related mortality is four times greater in women diagnosed during pregnancy or immediately postpartum.[8] In a study with patients with limited disease treated with adrenalectomy or adrenalectomy plus mitotane, fetal outcomes were good and overall survival was not affected by pregnancy compared to matched controls. None of the women in this study were treated with mitotane preconception or during pregnancy.[6]
- Given the poor prognosis, it has been suggested that surgical resection be considered first line, regardless of the trimester, and mitotane should be offered, even in tumors limited to the adrenal gland in this population.[6,8]
  - Complete tumor resection is the most efficient treatment. A laparoscopic or open approach may be used. Open surgery is typically recommended for limited disease as laparoscopic surgery is associated with a higher risk of developing recurrence, tumor rupture, or carcinomatosis.[6] In pregnancy, the laparoscopic approach may be preferred due to the advantages of shorter operative time, little interference to the abdominal cavity, and less bleeding. Carbon dioxide pneumoperitoneum which can occur secondary to gas insufflation in laparoscopic surgery can increase blood CO_2 partial pressure in pregnant patients and pose a potential threat to the fetus. The enlarged uterus may also pose a challenge in this approach.[5]

- If ACC is discovered in the first trimester, abortion for medical reasons may be discussed, especially for stage 3 or 4 disease.[8]
- Postoperatively, intravenous or oral hydrocortisone replacement is recommended to treat adrenal insufficiency.[5]
- Data in nonpregnant patients suggest mitotane treatment may prolong recurrence-free survival in ACC with radical resection. However, it is not recommended during pregnancy.[8]
- While there is a theoretical risk of disorders of sexual development in the fetus due to excess androgen production in ACC, there is little supporting evidence for this.[1]
- Case reports have described successful conception on mitotane and use during pregnancy without evidence of adrenal dysfunction in the fetus.[1] The suspicion that mitotane can cross the placenta comes from observations of the morphologically similar pesticide DDT, which is found in the cord blood of infants in DDT-exposed areas. In one case where elective abortion was performed at 21 weeks gestation, amniotic fluid and cord blood levels of mitotane were undetectable. Another case report detected similar levels of mitotane in cord blood to maternal serum and the newborn's ACTH level was significantly elevated yet blood cortisol was normal.[13] Given the lack of good evidence and long-term data regarding fetal exposure in utero, the current sentiment is that it should not be used during pregnancy but should be prescribed as soon as possible after delivery.[6]
- Mitotane is classified by the FDA as pregnancy category D. It has been detected in breast milk and hence breastfeeding is not recommended while on this medication.[14]

REFERENCES

1. Else T, Kim AC, Sabolch A, Raymond VM, Kandathil A, Caoili EM, et al. Adrenocortical Carcinoma. Endocrine Reviews. 2013;35(2): 282–326.
2. Eschler DC, Kogekar N, Pessah-Pollack R. Management of Adrenal Tumors in Pregnancy. Endocrinology and Metabolism Clinics of North America. 2015;44(2): 381–397.

3. Lacroix A. Clinical Presentation and Evaluation of Adrenocortical Tumors [Internet]. 2019 [cited 2021 Jan 21]. Available from: https://www.uptodate.com/contents/clinical-presentation-and-evaluation-of-adrenocortical-tumors#H11

4. Raffin-Sanson M-L, Abiven G, Ritzel K, Corbière PD, Cazabat L, Zaharia R, et al. Corticosurrénalome et grossesse. Annales d'Endocrinologie. 2016;77:139–147.

5. Zhang Y, Yuan Z, Qiu C, Li S, Zhang S, Fang Y. The Diagnosis and Treatment of Adrenocortical Carcinoma in Pregnancy: A Case Report. BMC Pregnancy and Childbirth. 2020;20(1):1–5.

6. Kiseljak-Vassiliades K, Bancos I, Hamrahian A, Habra M, Vaidya A, Levine AC, et al. American Association of Clinical Endocrinology Disease State Clinical Review on the Evaluation and Management of Adrenocortical Carcinoma in an Adult: A Practical Approach. Endocrine Practice. 2020;26(11):1366–1383.

7. Jairath A, Aulakh BS. Adrenocortical Carcinoma in Pregnancy: A Diagnostic Dilemma. Indian Journal of Urology. 2014 Jul;30(3):342–344.

8. Abiven-Lepage G, Coste J, Tissier F, Groussin L, Billaud L, Dousset B, et al. Adrenocortical Carcinoma and Pregnancy: Clinical and Biological Features and Prognosis. European Journal of Endocrinology. 2010 Nov;163(5):793–800.

9. Lekarev O, New MI. Adrenal Disease in Pregnancy. Best Practice & Research: Clinical Endocrinology & Metabolism. 2011;25(6):959–973.

10. Lindsay JR, Jonklaas J, Oldfield EH, Nieman LK. Cushing's Syndrome during Pregnancy: Personal Experience and Review of the Literature. Journal of Clinical Endocrinology & Metabolism. 2005 May 1;90(5):3077–3083.

11. Nolton WE, Lindheimer MD, Rueckert PA, Oparil S, Ehrlich EN. Diurnal Patterns and Regulation of Cortisol Secretion in Pregnancy. Journal of Clinical Endocrinology & Metabolism. 1980 Sep 1;51(3):466–472.

12. Morris LF, Park S, Daskivich T, Churchill BM, Rao CV, Lei Z, et al. Virilization of a Female Infant by a Maternal Adrenocortical Carcinoma. Endocrine Practice. 2011 Apr;17(2):E26–E31.

13. Tripto-Shkolnik L, Blumenfeld Z, Bronshtein M, Salmon A, Jaffe A. Pregnancy in a Patient with Adrenal Carcinoma Treated with Mitotane: A Case Report and Review of Literature. Journal of Clinical Endocrinology and Metabolism. 2013 Feb;98(2):443–447.

14. Bristol-Myers Squibb Company. Lysodren (Mitotane). U.S. Food and Drug Administration website: https://www.accessdata.fda.gov/drugsatfda_docs/label/2013/016885s025lbl.pdf. Revised Nov 2013. Accessed June 2021.

Adrenal insufficiency

JULIA C.W. LAKE

- Pregnancy is associated with significantly increased hypothalamic-pituitary-adrenal (HPA) axis activity, with serum cortisol and aldosterone levels multiple-fold higher than in the nonpregnant state.
- The diagnosis of adrenal insufficiency in pregnancy includes an 8 AM cortisol level <3.0 μg/dL or 250 μg cosyntropin-stimulated cortisol <25 μg/dL in the first trimester, <29 μg/dL in the second trimester, or <32 μg/dL in the third trimester.
- Hydrocortisone at a daily dose of 12–15 mg/m² of body surface area is the glucocorticoid

- of choice in pregnancy. Doses may need adjustment by a 20–40% increase in the second or third trimester.
- Stress dose intravenous hydrocortisone at a dose of 50–100 mg every 6–8 hours should be administered during the second stage of vaginal labor. Prior to cesarean section, a 100 mg intravenous stress dose of hydrocortisone should be administered.
- In patients with primary adrenal insufficiency, fludrocortisone doses may need to be increased during pregnancy.

EPIDEMIOLOGY

- The prevalence of primary adrenal insufficiency is estimated at 117–140 cases per million in predominantly Caucasian populations.[1,2]
- The incidence of primary adrenal insufficiency is 4.7–6.2 per million and cases are suspected to be on the rise.[1,2]
- The leading cause of primary adrenal insufficiency in the developed world is autoimmune adrenalitis (Addison's disease).
- Autoimmune adrenalitis has a female predominance, with the diagnosis most frequently made in the third through fifth decades of life.[3]
- In countries with a high prevalence of tuberculosis, tuberculosis adrenalitis is a major cause of primary adrenal insufficiency.[4]

- Secondary adrenal insufficiency is more common than primary adrenal insufficiency, with an estimated prevalence of 150–280 per million.[5]

PATHOPHYSIOLOGY

- Adrenal insufficiency is a nonspecific term used to describe the clinical syndrome of cortisol deficiency.
- Although uncommon, adrenal insufficiency may present insidiously during pregnancy with potentially grave consequences for both the mother and fetus.
- Perturbations in any of the three components of the HPA axis may lead to clinically evident adrenal insufficiency.

DOI: 10.1201/9781003027577-21

- Primary adrenal insufficiency is diagnosed when both mineralocorticoid and glucocorticoid production are deficient due to adrenal cortex dysfunction.
- Secondary and tertiary adrenal insufficiency may result from any process that interrupts pituitary adrenocorticotropic hormone (ACTH) or hypothalamic corticotropin-releasing hormone (CRH) secretion, respectively.
- The most common cause of central (secondary or tertiary) adrenal insufficiency is long-term exogenous corticosteroid use, leading to anterior pituitary corticotroph atrophy, diminished pituitary ACTH secretion, and subsequent adrenal cortex atrophy with diminished cortisol release. Secondary adrenal insufficiency is not associated with mineralocorticoid deficiency as the zona glomerulosa remains responsive to the action of the renin-angiotensin-aldosterone system (RAAS).[5]

Glucocorticoids and maternal adrenal function

- Pregnancy is associated with a state of markedly increased HPA axis function. Due to the hyperestrogenemia of pregnancy, hepatic production of corticosteroid-binding globulin (CBG) increases to double the prepregnancy values.
- Maternal ACTH levels rise gradually over the course of pregnancy. By weeks 33–37 of gestation, there is a mean 5-fold increase in ACTH levels over nonpregnant values and a dramatic 15-fold rise during labor.[6]
- Placental production of CRH and ACTH begins to rise starting in the seventh week of gestation, stimulating increases in maternal total and free cortisol levels.[7,8]
- These physiologic adaptations are associated with gradual increases in total serum and salivary free cortisol levels as pregnancy progresses.[9] By week 26 of gestation, a 3-fold increase in plasma cortisol is present.[10]
- Despite the significant rise in cortisol levels, pregnant women do not demonstrate the stigmata classically associated with Cushing's syndrome, such as ecchymoses, proximal muscle weakness, and dorsocervical adiposity.

- Prior theories have suggested that the anti-glucocorticoid effects of elevated progesterone levels during pregnancy lead to relatively inert cortisol actions.[11,12]
- Similarly, the physiologic cortisol elevation does not affect the developing fetus.
  - 11-β-hydroxysteroid dehydrogenase 2 (11β-HSD2) catalyzes the conversion of most of maternal cortisol to inert cortisone, thereby decreasing excess fetal glucocorticoid exposure, which could lead to intrauterine growth restriction and preeclampsia.[13]

Glucocorticoids and fetal adrenal function

- The fetal adrenal gland is derived from both mesoderm (cortex) and ectoderm (medulla). The primordia of the adrenal glands can be recognized by weeks 5–6 of gestation.[10–14] By weeks 7–8 of gestation, the mesodermal cells are infiltrated by sympathetic cells derived from neural crest tissue that will form the adrenal medulla.
- The fetal adrenal gland contains both a definitive zone, which later forms the adult zona glomerulosa, fasciculata, and reticularis, in addition to a much larger fetal zone. The fetal zone produces large amounts of inactive dehydroepiandrosterone (DHEA) and dehydroepiandrosterone-sulfate (DHEA-S) in comparison to cortisol due to a relative 3β-hydroxysteroid dehydrogenase (3β-HSD) deficiency and a predominance of DHEA sulfotransferase.[15]
- Fetal DHEA and DHEA-S are ultimately converted to estrogens by the placenta.[14,16]
- Glucocorticoids are produced by the fetus in the first trimester by transient expression of fetal 3β-HSD2, which reaches peak production between 8 and 9 months. The primary stimulus for fetal adrenal function is fetal pituitary ACTH.[17]
- Fetal HPA negative feedback is intact by the second half of gestation. Evidence for this is found in virilizing congenital adrenal hyperplasia (CAH), where it has been demonstrated that dexamethasone administration can inactivate placental 11β-HSD2.[18]

- Roughly two-thirds of fetal cortisol is derived from the fetal adrenal glands; the remaining one-third is derived from placental transfer.[10,19]

Mineralocorticoids

- Increased demands on maternal circulation during normal pregnancy are associated with changes in the RAAS. By full term in a normal pregnancy, the total systemic blood volume has increased by 40–45% to provide adequate perfusion to both the mother and the fetal-placental unit. Red blood cell mass increases by 20%. Plasma volume increases by 45–50% due to aldosterone-mediated sodium retention. Despite this, blood pressure falls due to increased vascular distensibility and reduced peripheral vascular resistance secondary to vasodilatory prostaglandins from the utero-placental unit.[20] Together, these changes reduce hematocrit by 15% at term, allowing for a reduction in the mass of red blood cells lost per any volume of blood loss during delivery and thus protection of oxygen-carrying capacity.[21]
- Plasma renin activity increases in the first trimester due to the presence of increased substrates produced by the liver under the effects of estrogen.[22] At full term, renin and angiotensin levels have increased 3- to 8-fold higher than the normal nonpregnant female range.[13,22,23] By the 38th week of gestation, there is a 10- to 20-fold increase in plasma aldosterone concentrations.[22,24] Despite this dramatic rise in aldosterone levels, the RAAS maintains normal physiologic responses to positional changes without occurrence of hypokalemia or hypernatremia.
- Pregnancy is associated with an increase in glomerular filtration rate (GFR) of 50% and thus an increase in the filtered sodium load.[13] Reduced urinary excretion of sodium before and after saline infusion suggests that pregnant women have an increased sodium requirement for homeostasis.[25]
- Progesterone levels increase in parallel with increases in plasma estradiol levels over the course of pregnancy. Progesterone acts as a mineralocorticoid receptor antagonist, displacing aldosterone from its renal receptors.[12] By near term, the human fetal adrenal gland is capable of aldosterone secretion due to development of the zona glomerulosa.[10,17]

DIAGNOSIS

Clinical presentation

- Most cases of primary adrenal insufficiency are diagnosed prior to pregnancy; however, the stress of labor may precipitate an adrenal crisis in a patient with undiagnosed primary adrenal insufficiency. A high degree of suspicion may be required to diagnose adrenal insufficiency during pregnancy as several symptoms are nonspecific and frequently occur during normal pregnancy.
- Evaluation for adrenal insufficiency is warranted in any pregnant woman presenting with subacute onset of fatigue, anorexia, weight loss, abdominal pain, orthostasis, hyperpigmentation, vomiting, hypoglycemia, hyperkalemia, or hyponatremia. A higher degree of suspicion is warranted in patients with preexisting autoimmune conditions such as type I diabetes mellitus or vitiligo.[26]
- Clinical presentation of adrenal insufficiency in pregnancy is often unclear:
  - Hyperkalemia may not be present in pregnant patients with primary adrenal insufficiency.
  - Hyponatremia is common during normal pregnancy.
  - Hyperpigmentation (melasma) is common during normal pregnancy. Of note, hyperpigmentation associated with excess pro-opiomelanocortin and ACTH in the setting of primary adrenal insufficiency usually manifests in areas of increased mechanical friction such as scars, knuckles, toes, and oral mucosa, whereas melasma of pregnancy only occurs in sun-exposed areas.[27]
  - Persistent vomiting associated with adrenal insufficiency may be mistaken for hyperemesis gravidarum, particularly in the first trimester.[26-28]
- In the setting of suspected secondary adrenal insufficiency, HPA axis assessment is warranted for women receiving 5 mg of prednisone daily or its equivalent for more than 3 weeks as this may lead to suppression of ACTH

levels with subsequent atrophy of the zona fasciculata.[29]

Laboratory assessment

- When clinical suspicion for adrenal insufficiency is high, immediate treatment with glucocorticoids is warranted due to the potentially grave consequences of delaying treatment. Obtaining cortisol and ACTH levels should not delay corticosteroid administration.
- Several complex changes occur in the HPA axis during pregnancy which ultimately lead to elevations in total plasma cortisol and CBG values.[13,30] These factors must be considered when interpreting the lab values of pregnant patients.
- Random early morning cortisol levels <3.0 µg/dl confirm the diagnosis of adrenal insufficiency if the patient demonstrates a classic clinical presentation.[31,32]
- Morning cortisol levels between 3 and 32 µg/dL should be interpreted with caution, especially in the second and third trimesters when they may appear falsely normal.[33] In these cases, formal dynamic testing of the HPA axis with a cosyntropin stimulation test is required.
  - A plasma cortisol value of <18 µg/dL 30 minutes after the administration of 250 µg of cosyntropin was previously suggested as a cutoff for the diagnosis of adrenal insufficiency during pregnancy.
  - Subsequent authors suggest using 30 µg/dL as a cutoff following a 250 µg cosyntropin stimulation test based upon previously reported 8 AM third trimester plasma cortisol levels and results from low-dose cosyntropin stimulation tests.[31]
  - More recent data suggest trimester-specific cosyntropin stimulation test cortisol cutoffs of 25 µg/dL in the first trimester, 29 µg/dL in the second trimester, and 32 µg/dL in the third trimester.[23,32,34]
- Insulin tolerance testing is contraindicated in pregnancy due to potential risks to the fetus when maternal blood glucose levels are <40 mg/dL. Similarly, the metyrapone stimulation test is not recommended during pregnancy due to the risk of precipitating adrenal crisis.

- Once cortisol deficiency is confirmed, differentiating between primary and secondary adrenal insufficiency with an ACTH level is the next step.
  - A plasma ACTH >100 pg/mL is consistent with primary adrenal insufficiency even in late pregnancy when levels are expected to be elevated.[13]
  - More than one measurement should be obtained as levels may fluctuate widely. The sample should be collected in a pre-chilled EDTA tube and transported on an ice bath.
  - Additional workup may be warranted based on clinical presentation. For instance, 21 hydroxylase antibodies, if present, should prompt assessment for autoimmune polyglandular syndromes, which may also include type I diabetes mellitus, autoimmune thyroid disease, pernicious anemia, and celiac disease.

TREATMENT

- Glucocorticoid replacement in primary and secondary adrenal insufficiency is not associated with teratogenicity or increased fetal loss.[35,36]
- Hydrocortisone is the preferred glucocorticoid replacement during pregnancy at a physiologic dose of 12–15 mg/m[2] of body surface area.[37] Two-thirds of the total hydrocortisone dose should be administered upon awakening and the remaining one-third should be dosed in the late afternoon to mimic normal diurnal variation. Some patients may prefer to take three daily doses but adherence may decrease with this regimen and no morbidity or mortality improvements have been proven as compared to twice-daily dosing.[38]
- Glucocorticoid doses do not typically need to be increased during early pregnancy. However, rises in CBG may lead to a higher hydrocortisone dosing requirement later in pregnancy. A common clinical approach is to increase hydrocortisone doses by 20–40% starting in the second or third trimester.[32]
- Determining whether glucocorticoid replacement is sufficient is based upon clinical parameters such as blood pressure, weight, and blood glucose levels each trimester.[32] ACTH, 24-hour

urinary free cortisol, and random cortisol levels should not be used to adjust dosing.[39,40]

- Under-replacement of glucocorticoid increases the risk for adrenal crisis. Over-replacement increases the risk of gestational diabetes, gestational hypertension, worsening of preexisting preeclampsia, weight gain, and, if chronic, an increased mortality due to cardiovascular disease.[41,42]
- Adrenal insufficiency requires increased glucocorticoid doses during labor.
  - Stress dose intravenous hydrocortisone 50–100 mg should be administered during the second stage of vaginal labor with subsequent doses determined on progress of labor.[23]
  - Prior to cesarean section, an intravenous 100 mg stress dose of hydrocortisone should be administered and continued at 6- to 8-hour intervals following delivery.[23]
  - Hydrocortisone is metabolized by placental 11β-HSD2, making excess glucocorticoid exposure to the fetus a highly improbable occurrence. Subsequent tapering over 48 hours to regular replacement doses should be sufficient to return to prepregnancy requirements without precipitation of a crisis.[27,32]
  - Less than 0.5% of absorbed glucocorticoid is excreted per liter of breast milk.[36]
- Fludrocortisone for patients with primary adrenal insufficiency is usually dosed at 0.1 mg daily in both pregnant and nonpregnant patients with doses ranging between 0.05 and 0.2 mg daily. The dose of mineralocorticoid may increase depending on serum potassium levels during pregnancy due to the anti-mineralocorticoid effects of progesterone but typically remains stable.[32]

REFERENCES

1. Lovas, Kristian, and Eystein S. Husebye. "High prevalence and increasing incidence of Addison's disease in Western Norway." Clin Endocrinol 56, no. 6 (2002): pp 787–791.
2. Laureti, Stefano, Luigi Vecchi, Fausto Santeusanio, and Alberto Falnori. "Is the prevalence of Addison's disease underestimated?" JCEM 84, no. 5 (1999): p 1762.
3. Kong, Marie-France, and William Jeffcoate. "Eighty-six cases of Addison's disease." Clin Endocrinol 41, no. 6 (1994): pp 757–761.
4. Soule, Steven. "Addison's disease in Africa: a teaching hospital experience." Clin Endocrinol 50, no. 1 (1999): pp. 115–120.
5. Nicolaides, NC et al. Adrenal Insufficiency. In: Feingold KR, Anawalt B, Boyce A et al., editors. Endotext [Internet]. South Dartmouth, MA: MDText.com, Inc.; (2000).
6. Carr, Bruce R., C. Richard Parker, James D. Madden, Paul C. MacDonald, and John C. Porter. "Maternal plasma adrenocorticotropin and cortisol relationships throughout human pregnancy." Am J Obstet Gynecol 139, no. 4 (1981): pp 416–422.
7. Ambroziak U, Agnieszka Kondracka, Zbigniew Bartoszewicz, Malgorzata Krasnodebska-Kiljanska, and Tomasz Bednarczuk. "The morning and late-night salivary cortisol ranges for healthy women may be used in pregnancy." Clin Endocrinol 83, no. 6 (2015): pp 774–778.
8. Dorr, Helmuth G., Andreas Heller, Hans T. Versmold, Wolfgang G. Sippell, Marion Herrmann, Frank Bidlingmaier, and Dieter Knorr. "Longitudinal study of progestins, mineralocorticoids, and glucocorticoids throughout human pregnancy." J Clin Endocrinol Metab 68, no. 5 (1989): pp 863–868.
9. Allolio, Bruno, Jochen Hoffmann, E. A. Linton, Werner Winkelmann, Martin Kusche, and Heinrich M. Schulte. "Diurnal salivary cortisol patterns during pregnancy and after delivery: relationship to plasma corticotrophin releasing-hormone." Clinical Endocrinol 33, no. 2 (1990): pp 279–289.
10. Winter, Jeremy, Richard A. Polin, William W. Fox, and Steven H. Abman. Fetal and Neonatal Adrenocortical Physiology. Elsevier Health Sciences (2004): pp 1915–1922.
11. Kajantie, Eero, Leo Dunkel, Ursula Turpeinen, Ulf-Hakan Stenman, Peter J. Wood, Mika Nuutila, and Sture Andersson. "Placental 11 β-hydroxysteroid dehydrogenase-2 and fetal cortisol/cortisone shuttle in small preterm infants." J Clin Endocrinol Metab 88, no. 1 (2003): pp 493–500.

12. Quinkler M., B. Meyer, C. Burnke-Vogt, C. Grossman, U., Gruber, W. Oelkers, S. Diederich, and V. Bahr. "Agonistic and antagonistic properties of progesterone metabolites at the human mineralocorticoid receptor." Eur J Endocrinol 146, no. 6 (2002): pp 789–799.

13. Lindsay John R, and Lynette K. Nieman. "The hypothalamic-pituitary-adrenal axis in pregnancy: challenges in disease detection and treatment." Endocr Rev 26, no. 6 (2005): pp 775–799.

14. Strauss III, Jerome, Fredrico Martinez, and Marianthi Kiriakidou. "Placental steroid hormone synthesis: unique features and unanswered questions." Biol Reprod 54, no. 2 (1996): pp 303–311.

15. Parker, CR. "Dehydroepiandrosterone and dehydroepiandrosterone sulfate production in the human adrenal during development and aging." Steroids 64 (1999): pp 640–647.

16. Geller DH, and Miller WL. Molecular development of the adrenal gland. In: Pescovitz Ora Hirsch and Erica A. Eugster, editors. Pediatric Endocrinology: Mechanisms, Manifestations, and Management. Section VIII Adrenal, chapter 36. Philadelphia, PA: Lippincott Williams & Wilkins; (2004): pp 561–572.

17. Mesiano, Sam. Endocrinology of human pregnancy and fetal-placental neuroendocrine development. In: Yen and Jaffe's Reproductive Endocrinology. Amsterdam: Elsevier; (2019): pp 256–284. Elsevier, USA.

18. Michel, David, and Maguelone G. Forest. "Prenatal treatment of congenital adrenal hyperplasia resulting from 21-hydroxylase deficiency." J Pediatr 105, no. 5 (1984): pp 799–803.

19. Otta Carolina Fux, Paula Szafryk de Mereshian, Gabriel Santino Iraci, and Maria Rosa Ojeda de Pruneda. "Pregnancies associated with primary adrenal insufficiency." Fertil Steril 90, no. 4 (2008): pp 1199.e17–1199.e20.

20. Bird, Ian M, Lubo Zhand, and Ronald R. Magness. "Possible mechanisms underlying pregnancy-induced changes in uterine artery endothelial function." Am J Physiol Regul Integr Comp Physiol 284, no. 2 (2003): pp R245–R258.

21. Soma-Pillay, Priya, Catherine Nelson-Piercy, Heli Tolppanen, and Alexandre Mebazaa. "Physiological changes in pregnancy." Cardiovasc J Afr 27, no. 2 (2016): p 89 doi:10.5830/CVJA-2016-021.

22. Wilson, Maxim, Alberto Morganti, Ioannis Zervoudakis, RL Letcher, BM Romney, P Von Oeyon, S Papera, Jean E Sealey, and John H Laragh. "Blood pressure, the renin-aldosterone system and sex steroids throughout normal pregnancy." Am J Med 68, no. 1 (1980): pp 97–104.

23. Langlois, Fabienne, ST Dawn, and Maria Fleseriu. "Update on adrenal insufficiency: diagnosis and management in pregnancy." Curr Opin Endocrinol Diabetes Obes 24, no. 3 (2017): pp184–192.

24. Sims Ethan, AH, and Kermit E. Krantz. "Serial studies of renal function during pregnancy and the puerperium in normal women." J Clin Investig 37, no. 12 (1958): pp 1764–1774.

25. Weinberger, Myron H, Norman J. Kramer, Clarence E. Grim, and Loren P. Petersen. "The effect of posture and saline loading on plasma renin activity and aldosterone concentration in pregnant, nonpregnant and estrogen treated women." J Clin Endocrinol Metab 44, no. 1 (1977): pp 69–77.

26. George, LD, R Selvaraju, K Reddy, TV Stout, and LD KE Premawardhana. "Vomiting and hyponatremia in pregnancy." BLOG-Int J Obstet Gy 107, no. 6 (2000): pp 808–809.

27. Lebbe M, and Arlt W. What is the best diagnostic and therapeutic management strategy for an Addison patient during pregnancy? Clin Endocrinol 78 (2013): pp 497–502.

28. Seaward, PG, RF Guidozzi, and EWW Sonnendecker. "Addisonian crisis in pregnancy. Case report." BJOG 96, no. 11 (1989): pp 1348–1350.

29. McKenna David S, Glynn M Wittber, Nagaraja HN, and Phillip Samuels. "The effects of repeat doses of antenatal corticosteroids on maternal adrenal function." Am J Obstet Gynecol 183, no. 3 (2000): pp 669–673.

30. Petraglia Felice, Paul E Sawchenko, Jean Rivier, and Wylie Vale. "Evidence for local stimulation of ACTH secretion by

corticotropin-releasing factor in human placenta." Nature 328 (1987): pp 717–719.

31. Grinspoon Steven K, and BM Biller. "Clinical review 62: Laboratory assessment of adrenal insufficiency." J Clin Endocrin Metab 79, no. 4 (1994): pp 923–931.

32. Bornstein Stefan R, Bruno Allolio, Wiebke Arlt, Andreas Barthel, Andrew Don-Wauchope, Gary D. Hammer, Eystein S Husebye et al. "Diagnosis and treatment of primary adrenal insufficiency: an Endocrine Society Clinical Practice guideline." J Clin Endocrinol Metab 101, no. 2 (2016): pp 364–389.

33. Nolten WE, MD Lindheimer, S Oparil, PA Rueckert, and EN Ehrlich. "Desoxycorticosterone in normal pregnancy. II Cortisol-dependent fluctuations in free plasma desoxycorticosterone." Am J Obstet Gynecol 133, no. 6 (1979): pp 644–648.

34. Fleseriu, Maria, Ibrahim A. Hashim, Niki Karavitaki, Shlomo Melmed, M. Hassan Murad, Roberto Salvatori, and Mary H. Samuels. "Hormonal replacement in hypopituitarism in adults: an Endocrine Society Clinical Practice guideline." J Clin Endocrinol Metab 101, no. 11 (2016): pp 3888–3921.

35. Walsh, Sadie D, and FR Clark. "Pregnancy in patients on long-term corticosteroid therapy." Scott Med J 12, no. 9 (1967): pp 302–306.

36. Sidhu Rajinder, K, and DF Hawkins. "Prescribing in pregnancy-corticosteroids." Clin Obstet Gynaecol 8 (1981): pp 383–404.

37. Yuen, Kevin CJ, Lindsay E Chong, and Christian A Koch. "Adrenal insufficiency in pregnancy: challenging issues in diagnosis and management." Endocrine 44 (2013): pp 283–292.

38. Groves, RW, GC Toms, BJ Houghton, and Monson, JP. (1988). "Corticosteroid replacement therapy: twice or thrice daily?" J R Soc Med 81, no. 9 (1988): pp 514–516.

39. Feek, CM, JG Ratcliffe, J Seth, CE Gray, AD Toft, and WK Irvine. "Patterns of plasms cortisol and ACTH concentrations in patients with Addison's disease treated with conventional corticosteroid replacement." Clin Endocrinol 14, no. 5 (1981): pp 451–458.

40. Hahner Stephanie, and Allolio Bruno. "Therapeutic management of adrenal insufficiency." Best Pract Res Clin Endocrinol Metab 23, no. 2 (2009): pp 167–179.

41. Anand, Gurpreet, and Felix Beuschlein. "Fertility, pregnancy and lactation in women with adrenal insufficiency." Eur J Endocrinol 178, no. 2 (2018): pp R45–R53.

42. Bergthorsdottir Ragnhildur, Maria Leonsson-Zachrisson, Anders Oden, and Gudmendur Johansson. "Premature mortality in patients with Addison's disease: a population-based study." JCEM 91, no. 12 (2006): 4849–4853.

4g

Congenital adrenal hyperplasia

RESHMITHA RADHAKRISHNAN AND THARANI RAJESWARAN

KEY POINTS

- Adrenal steroidogenesis entails the processes of cholesterol conversion into glucocorticoids, mineralocorticoids, and androgens.
- Steroid hormones play a critical role in stress responses, salt and water regulation, and sexual and reproductive development.
- Congenital adrenal hyperplasia (CAH) is a group of autosomal recessive disorders which are characterized by impaired steroid synthesis.
- The most common cause of CAH is a deficiency of the enzyme 21-hydroxylase caused by mutation in the *CYP21A2* gene.[1,2] It accounts for more than 95% of CAH.

- Other forms include 3β-hydroxysteroid dehydrogenase deficiency associated with mutation in the 3β-hydroxysteroid dehydrogenase (3β-HSD2) gene and 11β-hydroxylase deficiency due to a mutation in the 11β-hydroxylase (*CYP11B1*) gene.
- Patients with classic CAH require treatment with glucocorticoids and mineralocorticoids lifelong.
- Patients with nonclassic CAH may require steroids prior to conception to induce ovulation, however, usually do not require continuation of glucocorticoids during pregnancy.

EPIDEMIOLOGY

- Neonatal screening studies approximate that the incidence of CAH in the world is 1:14,000 to 1:18,000 people. In the United States and Europe alone, CAH affects 1:10,000 to 1:15,000 individuals.[3]
- The incidence is higher among certain populations. Among Ashkenazi Jews and the Yupik Eskimos, the occurrence is as high as 1 in 282 individuals.[4]
- Classic CAH is present in approximately 1 in 16,000 and nonclassic CAH in 1 in 600 individuals, making it one of the most common recessive genetic disorders.[5]

PATHOPHYSIOLOGY

- Corticotropin-releasing hormone (CRH) produced by the hypothalamus stimulates the pituitary gland to produce adrenocorticotropic hormone (ACTH).
- ACTH then stimulates the synthesis of cortisol by the adrenal cortex.
- The adrenal cortex is divided into three zones:
  - Zona glomerulosa secretes mineralocorticoids
  - Zona fasciculata secretes glucocorticoids
  - Zona reticularis secretes sex steroids
- Various mutations occurring in the *CYP21A2* gene encoding 21-hydroxylase affect the severity of CAH.

DOI: 10.1201/9781003027577-22

- In classic CAH, there is largely no enzyme activity. This results in deficiency of cortisol and aldosterone. Milder forms of CAH have partial enzyme activity, resulting in milder or negligible cortisol deficiency.
- 21-hydroxylase converts 17-hydroxyprogesterone (17-OHP) to 11-deoxycortisol, a precursor of cortisol. 21-hydroxylase also converts progesterone to deoxycorticosterone, a precursor of aldosterone.
- 21-hydroxylase deficiency leads to a decrease in production of cortisol and, as a result of negative feedback, an increase in release of ACTH by the pituitary gland. A surge in ACTH increases synthesis of 17-OHP and progesterone, which then serve as substrates for increased androgen production.

DIAGNOSIS

- Classic CAH is diagnosed early in childhood, while the milder form, nonclassic CAH, is typically diagnosed in adolescence or adulthood.
- Classic CAH, which can be further classified into simple virilizing and salt-wasting forms, is diagnosed in infancy.[6]
- Nonclassic CAH can present with hirsutism, temporal balding, and menstrual irregularities and therefore, is usually diagnosed prior to pregnancy.[7] Diagnosis should be made with an 8 AM 17-OHP level ideally drawn during the follicular phase, as ovulation can normally increase these levels.
  - A morning 17-OHP value of <200 ng/dL makes the diagnosis extremely unlikely.
  - An 8 AM 17-OHP >1000 ng/dL confirms the diagnosis.
  - If 17-OHP is between 200 and 1000 ng/dL, cosyntropin stimulation testing is recommended.
  - If cosyntropin stimulation testing is performed, a 17-OHP level >1000 ng/dL is consistent with the diagnosis.

TREATMENT

- Although some women with nonclassic CAH require treatment with steroids prior to pregnancy to induce ovulation, chronic steroid use or steroid use during pregnancy is not typically necessary.

- All patients with classic CAH require lifelong treatment with glucocorticoids and mineralocorticoids. Pregnant women with classic CAH should continue treatment with hydrocortisone or prednisolone and fludrocortisone throughout their pregnancy.
- If symptoms of adrenal insufficiency develop during pregnancy, the glucocorticoid dose can be increased 20–40%, starting in the 24th week of gestation.[8]
- Before delivery, an additional dose of 25–50 mg of hydrocortisone can be considered.
- Glucocorticoids that cross the placenta (e.g., dexamethasone) are not recommended.
  - However, if there is a positive history of CAH in a prior pregnancy or if both partners are heterozygous for a known mutation, treatment with dexamethasone may be indicated to decrease the risk of virilization of a female fetus.
  - Pregnancies at risk for fetal development of CAH need to be treated by 6 weeks after conception before virilization of female genitalia begins. As the formation of male genitalia is not affected by CAH, dexamethasone should not be part of prenatal treatment.
  - Treatment with dexamethasone is considered to be experimental as the long-term risks of treatment on the fetus and mother are largely unknown, but studies have shown that use of dexamethasone reduces genital virilization of 46XX fetuses.[9–14]

REFERENCES

1. White PC, New MI, Dupont B. HLA-linked congenital adrenal hyperplasia results from a defective gene encoding a cytochrome P-450 specific for steroid 21-hydroxylation. Proc Natl Acad Sci USA. 1984;81(23):7505–7509.
2. Krone N, Dhir V, Ivison HE, Arlt W. Congenital adrenal hyperplasia and P450 oxidoreductase deficiency. Clin Endocrinol (Oxf). 2007;66(2):162–172.
3. Milyani AA, Al-Agha AE, Al-Zanbagi M. Initial presentations and associated clinical findings in patients with classical congenital adrenal hyperplasia. J Pediatr Endocrinol Metab. 2018 Jun 27;31(6):671–673.
4. Pang S, Murphey W, Levine LS, et al. A pilot newborn screening for congenital adrenal

hyperplasia in Alaska. J Clin Endocrinol Metab 1982;55:413.

5. Speiser PW, Dupont BO, Rubinstein P, Piazza A, Kastelan A, New MI. High frequency of nonclassical steroid 21-hydroxylase deficiency. Obstet Gynecol Surv. 1986;41(4):244–245.

6. White PC, Speiser PW. Congenital adrenal hyperplasia due to 21-hydroxylase deficiency. Endocr Rev. 2000;21(3):245–291.

7. Kohn B, Levine LS, Pollack MS, Pang S, Lorenzen F, Levy D, Lerner AJ, Rondanini GF, Dupont B, New MI. Late-onset steroid 21-hydroxylase deficiency: a variant of classical congenital adrenal hyperplasia. J Clin Endocrinol Metab. 1982;55(5):817–827.

8. Bornstein SR, Allolio B, Arlt W, Barthel A, Don-Wauchope A, Hammer GD, Husebye ES, Merke DP, Murad MH, Stratakis CA, Torpy DJ. Diagnosis and treatment of primary adrenal insufficiency: an Endocrine Society Clinical Practice guideline. J Clin Endocrinol Metab. 2016;101(2):364–389.

9. Mercè Fernández-Balsells M, Muthusamy K, Smushkin G, Lampropulos JF, Elamin MB, Abu Elnour NO, Elamin KB, Speiser et al. Guidelines on congenital adrenal hyperplasia. J Clin Endocrinol Metab, 2018;103(11):4043–4088.

10. Agrwal N, Gallegos-Orozco JF, Lane MA, Erwin PJ, Montori VM, Murad MH. Prenatal dexamethasone use for the prevention of virilization in pregnancies at risk for classical congenital adrenal hyperplasia because of 21-hydroxylase (CYP21A2) deficiency: a systematic review and meta-analyses. Clin Endocrinol (Oxf). 2010;73(4):436–444.

11. Németh S, Riedl S, Kriegshäuser G, Baumgartner-Parzer S, Concolino P, Neocleous V, Phylactou LA, Borucka-Mankiewicz M, Onay H, Tukun A, Oberkanins C. Reverse-hybridization assay for rapid detection of common CYP21A2 mutations in dried blood spots from newborns with elevated 17-OH progesterone. Clin Chim Acta. 2012;414:211–214.

12. Carmichael SL, Shaw GM, Ma C, Werler MM, Rasmussen SA, Lammer EJ. National Birth Defects Prevention Study. Maternal corticosteroid use and orofacial clefts. Am J Obstet Gynecol. 2007;197:585(6):e1–7.

13. New MI, Carlson A, Obeid J, Marshall I, Cabrera MS, Goseco A, Lin-Su K, Putnam AS, Wei JQ, Wilson RC. Prenatal diagnosis for congenital adrenal hyperplasia in 532 pregnancies. J Clin Endocrinol Metab. 2001;86(12):5651–5657.

14. Pole JD, Mustard CA, To T, Beyene J, Allen AC. Antenatal steroid therapy for fetal lung maturation: is there an association with childhood asthma? J Asthma. 2009;46(1):47–52.

Adrenal emergencies: Adrenal crisis

JULIA C.W. LAKE

KEY POINTS

- Adrenal crisis is defined as an acute deterioration in health status in the setting of adrenal insufficiency associated with absolute hypotension (systolic blood pressure <100 mmHg) or relative hypotension with features that resolve within 1–2 hours after parenteral glucocorticoid administration.
- Laboratory assessment should never delay administration of glucocorticoids in suspected adrenal crisis.
- Both vaginal delivery and cesarean section require stress dose corticosteroids to prevent precipitation of adrenal crisis in those with known underlying adrenal insufficiency as well as in those without prior diagnosis of adrenal insufficiency but with suspected impending adrenal crisis.
- Rapid administration of 100 mg of intravenous hydrocortisone with repeat doses of 50 mg given every 6 hours thereafter and 1 L of intravenous normal saline over the first hour is the standard of care for treating adrenal crisis.
- Patient education regarding adrenal crisis prevention with emphasis placed on stress doses should be provided in writing to each patient with adrenal insufficiency.

EPIDEMIOLOGY

- The estimated prevalence of adrenal insufficiency in pregnant women is 5.5/100,000, with rates steadily rising.[1]
- Six to eight percent of patients with adrenal insufficiency experience an adrenal crisis annually.[2]
- Prior to the advent of hormonal substitution therapy in the 1950s, Addison's disease was associated with such a high maternal mortality of 35–45% that women who carried the diagnosis were discouraged from pursuing pregnancy.[3] The use of physiologic, and when appropriate, supraphysiologic doses of glucocorticoid and mineralocorticoid replacement has vastly improved maternal and fetal outcomes.[4]
- Despite modern advances, maternal mortality is still significantly higher in patients with primary adrenal insufficiency than in the general population (OR 22.30, 95% CI 6.82–72.96). This increased mortality is predominantly due to postpartum infection and venous thromboembolic phenomena.[1] Adrenal crisis during delivery or immediately thereafter is a commonly cited source of increased mortality in women with adrenal insufficiency, which can be avoided altogether if preventive management is performed appropriately.

DOI: 10.1201/9781003027577-23

PATHOPHYSIOLOGY

- Glucocorticoids act to increase blood pressure via two primary mechanisms:
  - In the vascular smooth muscle, they increase sensitivity to angiotensin II and catecholamines.
  - Simultaneously, they reduce nitric oxide-mediated endothelial dilatation.[5]
- In the kidney, glucocorticoids act to increase sodium retention and potassium loss via the mineralocorticoid receptor in the distal nephron.[6] Absence of these glucocorticoid-induced vasoactive and renal actions leads to hypotension, hyponatremia, and hyperkalemia.
- Cortisol suppresses inflammatory cytokines; the absence of this inhibition leads to malaise, anorexia, and fever. The lack of inhibition of inflammatory cytokines also leads to altered immune-cell populations with eosinophilia, neutropenia, and lymphocytosis seen in glucocorticoid-deficient patients.
- Gluconeogenesis is reduced in the setting of glucocorticoid deficiency, leading to hypoglycemia.
- The clinical manifestations of adrenal crisis may occur as soon as a few hours following the onset of cortisol deficiency as the circulating half-life of cortisol is 90 minutes.[7]
- Fetal glucocorticoid levels may affect maternal glucocorticoid levels. After the 33rd week of gestation, fetal adrenal cortisol production increases and maternal contribution decreases. In this setting, trans-placental passage of glucocorticoids from the fetus to the mother may have a protective effect in preventing adrenal crisis during delivery and in the immediate postnatal period.

DIAGNOSIS

- A widely accepted definition of an adrenal crisis is "an acute deterioration in health status associated with absolute hypotension (systolic blood pressure <100 mmHg) or relative hypotension (systolic blood pressure >20 mmHg lower than usual) with features that resolve within 1–2 hours after parenteral glucocorticoid administration."[7]

- Precipitants of adrenal crisis
  - Gastrointestinal infection is the most common precipitant of adrenal crisis for both pregnant and nonpregnant patients with adrenal insufficiency.[8]
  - Urinary tract infections are common triggers during pregnancy.
  - Hyperemesis gravidarum may lead to a crisis if the patient is not fully absorbing oral hydrocortisone.
  - Nonadherence to glucocorticoid replacement therapy or under-dosing, particularly in the second and third trimesters when requirements increase, may also precipitate an adrenal crisis.
  - Other potential triggers include hemorrhage, injury, and psychosocial stressors.[9]
  - Delivery itself may precipitate a crisis if the patient does not receive stress dose glucocorticoids prior to and throughout delivery. ACTH levels increase 15-fold during delivery, providing further evidence that stress dose glucocorticoids are essential during this period.[10]
- Random early morning cortisol levels <3.0 µg/dl confirm the diagnosis of adrenal insufficiency if the patient demonstrates a classic clinical presentation (see Chapter 4f).[11,12]
- Morning cortisol levels between 3 and 32 µg/dL should be interpreted with caution, especially in the second and third trimesters when they may appear falsely normal.[12,13]
- Trimester-specific 250 µg cosyntropin stimulation test cortisol cutoffs of 25 µg/dL in the first trimester, 29 µg/dL in the second trimester, and 32 µg/dL in the third trimester should only be used in nonstressed patients.[8,12] In general, cortisol levels must be interpreted with caution, as they are expected to rise dramatically in the setting of infection, illness, or stress.[14] It should also be noted that a cosyntropin stimulation test will not rule out acute central adrenal insufficiency due to recent pituitary dysfunction, as otherwise unaffected adrenal glands are expected to retain the ability to respond to cosyntropin for several months.
- Laboratory assessment should not delay administration of glucocorticoids in the setting of an adrenal crisis or suspected adrenal crisis.

TREATMENT

- Rapid administration of 100 mg hydrocortisone as an intravenous bolus with repeat doses of 50 mg given every 6 hours thereafter in addition to ≥1 L of intravenous normal saline over the first hour is the standard of care in the setting of suspected or confirmed adrenal crisis.[7]
- Treatment of the precipitating cause is a priority as it helps reduce subsequent events.
- Hydrocortisone at ≥50 mg has the equivalent of ≥0.1 mg of fludrocortisone and will provide sufficient mineralocorticoid activity such that fludrocortisone is not required during stress dosing.
- If hydrocortisone is not available, 4 mg intravenous dexamethasone is given every 24 hours or 25 mg prednisolone given as a bolus and followed by two 25 mg doses for a total of 75 mg in the first 24 hours may be used.[7] As these corticosteroids do not have enough mineralocorticoid activity, fludrocortisone should be continued.
- Intravenous dextrose may be required for hypoglycemia related to adrenal insufficiency.
- Patients and their family members should be educated regarding adrenal crisis prevention with an emphasis placed on the rationale for dose adjustments, the circumstances under which stress dosing is required, and when to seek emergency medical care. Discussion, instructions, and information provided to the patient should include the following:
  - Doses of hydrocortisone should be doubled if the patient's temperature exceeds 38°C and tripled if their temperature exceeds 39°C.[15]
  - Patients should receive a prescription for a one-time stress dose of intramuscular (IM) hydrocortisone 100 mg. A demonstration on how to properly administer the hydrocortisone intramuscularly will help ensure the patient can use it successfully under stressful circumstances. Patients should also seek emergency medical care any time the IM stress dose is deemed necessary.
  - All patients with adrenal insufficiency should be counseled on wearing a medical alert bracelet or necklace with detailed instructions on stress-related dose requirements. If the electronic medical record allows problem lists to be categorized in order of importance, adrenal insufficiency should be placed near the top with an easily identifiable note that the patient will require stress dose corticosteroids if critically ill.[7]
  - Pregnant patients who suspect that an adrenal crisis is imminent should seek immediate emergency care.

REFERENCES

1. Schneiderman, M., N. Czuzoj-Shulman, A. R. Spence, and H. A. Abenhain. "Maternal and neonatal outcomes of pregnancies in women with Addison's disease: a population-based cohort study on 7.7 million births." *BJOG: An International Journal of Obstetrics and Gynaecology* 124, no. 11 (2017): 1772–1779.
2. Rushworth, R. Louise, David J. Torpy, and Henrik Falhammer. "Adrenal crises: perspectives and research directions." *Endocrine* 55, no. 2 (2017): 336–345.
3. Brent, Florence. "Addison's disease and pregnancy." *The American Journal of Surgery* 79, no. 5 (1950): 645–652.
4. Remde, H., K. Zopf, J. Schwander, and M. Quinkler. "Fertility and pregnancy in primary adrenal insufficiency in Germany." *Hormone and Metabolic Research* 48, no. 5 (2016): 301–311.
5. Walker, Brian R., Alan. A. Connacher, David J. Webb, and Christopher R.W. Edwards. "Glucocorticoids and blood pressure: a role for the cortisol/cortisone shuttle in the control of vascular tone in man." *Clinical Science* 83, no. 2 (1992): 171–178.
6. Fraser, Robert, David L. Davies, and John McConnell. "Hormones and hypertension." *Clinical Endocrinology* 31, no. 6 (1989): 701–746.
7. Rushworth R., Louise, David J. Torpy, and Henrik Falhammar. "Adrenal crisis." *NEJM* 381, no. 9 (2019): 852–861.
8. Hahner, Stephanie, Christina Spinnler, Martin Fassnacht, Stephanie Burger-Stritt, Katharina Lang, Danijela Milovanovic, Felix Beuschlein, Holger S. Willenberg, Marcus Quinkler, and Bruno Allolio. "High Incidence of adrenal crisis in educated patients with

chronic adrenal insufficiency: a prospective study." *JCEM* 100, no. 2 (2015): 407–416.

9. McFarlane, C. N., and L. H. Truelove. "Addison's disease in pregnancy." *BJOG: An International Journal of Obstetrics & Gynaecology* 64, no. 6 (1957): 891–897.

10. Petraglia, Felice, Paul E. Sawchenko, Jean Rivier, and Wylie Vale. "Evidence for local stimulation of ACTH secretion by corticotropin-releasing factor in human placenta." *Nature* 328 (1987): 717–719.

11. Grinspoon Steven, K., and B. M. Biller. "Clinical review 62: Laboratory assessment of adrenal insufficiency." *Journal of Clinician Endocrinology & Metabolism* 79, no. 4 (1994): 923–931.

12. Suri, Daesman, Jill Moran, Judith U. Hibbard, Kristen Kasza, and Roy E. Weiss. "Assessment of adrenal reserve in pregnancy: defining the normal response to the adrenocorticotropin stimulation test."

Journal of Clinician Endocrinology & Metabolism 91, no. 10 (2006): 3866–3872.

13. Nolten, W. E., M. D. Lindheimer, S. Oparil, P. A. Rueckert, and E. N. Ehrlich. "Desoxycorticosterone in normal pregnancy. II Cortisol-dependent fluctuations in free plasma desoxycorticosterone." *American Journal of Obstetrics & Gynecology* 133, no. 6 (1979): 644–648.

14. Cooper, Mark Stuart, and Paul Michael Stewart. "Adrenal insufficiency in critical illness." *Journal of Intensive Care Medicine* 22, no. 6 (2007): 348–362.

15. Bornstein, Stefan R, Bruno Allolio, Wiebke Arlt, Andreas Barthel, Andrew Don-Wauchope, Gary D. Hammer, Eystein S. Husebye et al. "Diagnosis and treatment of primary adrenal insufficiency: an Endocrine Society clinical practice guideline." *Journal of Clinician Endocrinology & Metabolism* 101, no. 2 (2016): 364–389.

CHAPTER 5

Pituitary

Pituitary incidental adenomas

JESSICA PERINI

KEY POINTS

- Pituitary incidental adenomas (also called incidentalomas) are lesions located in the pituitary gland noted on imaging done for symptoms unrelated to pituitary hormone function.
- Microincidentalomas are lesions <1 cm whereas macroincidentalomas are lesions ≥1 cm.
- Pituitary incidentalomas may be nonfunctional or functional, producing excess amounts of a pituitary hormone.
- Determining whether a pituitary tumor is functional may be difficult during pregnancy.

- due to physiologic changes in some pituitary hormones during the gestational period.
- Incidentalomas may, by mass effect or by hormonal feedback, suppress pituitary hormone production.
- All patients with incidentalomas abutting the optic nerves or chiasm should undergo formal visual field testing, even in the absence of visual symptoms.
- Treatment for pituitary incidentalomas varies and includes observation, medications, or surgical resection, depending upon the tumor type and behavior.

EPIDEMIOLOGY

- In the nonpregnant population, pituitary incidentalomas can be found in up to 38% of imaging studies, with rates varying based on imaging technique, patient age, and other factors.[1]
- The incidence of pituitary incidentalomas is unclear in the pregnant population but may be higher than that in the general population due to the physiologic enlargement of the pituitary by 2- to 3-fold during pregnancy. Often this enlargement is misclassified as a pituitary adenoma.
- Pituitary incidentalomas are most commonly nonfunctional when found during pregnancy, as functional tumors often lead to infertility.[2]

PATHOPHYSIOLOGY

- Enlargement of the pituitary occurs physiologically during pregnancy, mainly due to the enlargement of lactotrophs. The size of the pituitary may increase up to 3-fold in normal pregnancy, returning to normal size within months after delivery.
- Prolactinomas
  - Microprolactinomas do not typically increase in size during pregnancy.
  - Pregnancy is associated with significant tumor growth of macroprolactinomas in up to 30% of cases.[3]
- Most other functional pituitary tumors do not increase in size during or due to pregnancy.

DOI: 10.1201/9781003027577-25

- Pregnancy does not typically lead to an increase in the size of nonfunctional pituitary adenomas; however, the physiologic enlargement of the pituitary gland, in addition to the presence of a previous tumor, may lead to new visual symptoms or headache.[2]
- Determining whether a pituitary incidentaloma is functional may be difficult, as pituitary hormones are often elevated due to physiologic changes of pregnancy.
- In normal pregnancy
  - Prolactin levels may rise to 300 ng/mL or more (nonpregnant normal: <25 ng/mL).
  - Growth hormone (GH) levels are elevated due to estrogen effects and placental GH.
  - Cortisol, adrenocorticotropic hormone (ACTH), and corticotropin-releasing hormone (CRH) are altered due to estrogen effects on cortisol-binding globulin (CBG), decreased clearance of cortisol, and production of CRH from the placenta, fetal membranes, and decidua.[4]

DIAGNOSIS

- When a pituitary mass is found incidentally during pregnancy, evaluation is necessary to determine whether the lesion is
  - Causing mass effect leading to visual field cuts or damage or risk to surrounding areas
  - Changing or enlarging over time
  - Hyperfunctioning and likely to cause harm to the pregnancy
  - Causing partial or complete hypopituitarism
- Imaging
  - The best imaging modality is MRI with pituitary protocol. In pregnancy, this is usually performed without gadolinium.
  - MRI can demonstrate the presence of impingement on or abutment of the optic chiasm.
  - MRI may show mass effect on surrounding areas of the brain that could cause harm for the patient (e.g. occlusion of vessels).
- Formal visual field testing is necessary if there is any optic chiasm or optic nerve involvement or visual symptoms.
- A thorough history and physical exam should be performed to assess for signs and symptoms of hormone dysfunction.

- Lab evaluation for hyperfunctioning
  - Prolactinoma
    - Diagnosing a prolactinoma during pregnancy is difficult, as prolactin levels rise significantly during normal pregnancy.
    - Many labs provide reference ranges for prolactin levels during pregnancy into the 300 ng/mL range, but not commonly >400; thus, prolactin levels >400 in the presence of a pituitary incidentaloma may suggest a prolactinoma.
    - Macroprolactinomas are the only type of pituitary tumor that are expected to increase in size during pregnancy; thus, these require special attention and close monitoring (see Chapter 5d).[5]
  - ACTH-producing tumor (Cushing's disease)
    - Diagnosis of Cushing's syndrome in pregnancy is described in Chapter 4d.
    - ACTH-producing pituitary tumors warrant treatment during pregnancy, as excess cortisol can increase morbidity and mortality.
  - TSH-producing tumor
    - Measure TSH, free T4, and total T4.
    - T4 levels significantly above normal range for gestational period with TSH that is elevated or inappropriately normal (unsuppressed TSH) is indicative of a TSHoma.
    - TSHomas warrant treatment during pregnancy, as hyperthyroidism can significantly complicate the pregnancy.
  - Growth hormone-secreting tumor (acromegaly)
    - Measurement of IGF-1 is the first step in diagnosing acromegaly.
    - IGF-1 is commonly elevated during normal pregnancy in the absence of acromegaly.
    - If acromegaly is suspected, observation through the pregnancy is generally acceptable (see Chapter 5b).[5]
  - LH or FSH-producing tumor:
    - Measurement of LH, FSH, and estradiol is not helpful or necessary during pregnancy.
- Lab evaluation for hypopituitarism
  - Central adrenal insufficiency

- For diagnostic evaluation, see Chapter 4f.
- Central hypothyroidism
  - Free or total T4 below normal range for gestational period with TSH that is low or inappropriately normal (not elevated) is indicative of central hypothyroidism.
  - Free or total T4 below normal range for gestational period with TSH that is elevated is indicative of primary hypothyroidism. Untreated primary hypothyroidism can lead to hypertrophy of the thyrotrophs of the pituitary and appear as a mass on pituitary imaging.
- No other hormonal evaluation for hypopituitarism is needed during pregnancy, although further workup may be performed postpartum.

TREATMENT

- Prolactinoma (see Chapter 5d)
  - Treatment is generally not advised if pregnancy is progressing appropriately, if the pituitary tumor is <1 cm, and if there is no involvement of the optic chiasm.
  - Visual field testing is necessary if the patient is experiencing visual symptoms or if the mass is known to involve the optic chiasm.
  - If the mass is a macroadenoma, significant growth may occur in up to 21% of cases; thus, closer monitoring is advised[3]:
    - Visual field testing every 1–3 months during pregnancy
    - Repeat MRI if headaches or visual defects develop or progress
  - Treatment can be initiated after careful consideration and discussion with the patient if the tumor growth is leading to symptoms and/or is rapid.
  - Treatment involves either use of dopamine agonist therapy or surgery.
    - Dopamine agonists may be safer for the patient and fetus than surgery, but data regarding the use of these drugs long-term through pregnancy are limited.
    - Although there are more data regarding the safety of bromocriptine in

pregnancy, cabergoline appears to be equally safe. Rates of adverse outcomes in pregnancy from either drug are similar to those in the general population.[3]
  - Despite similar safety profiles with bromocriptine and cabergoline in treatment of prolactinomas during pregnancy and despite the generally greater efficacy of cabergoline to reduce the size of a prolactinoma and prolactin levels, some countries do not approve the use of cabergoline in pregnancy.
- A dopamine agonist should be started at the lowest dose with prolactin level measured 2 weeks after initiation.
  - If the prolactin level is not declining, the dose should be increased in small increments, with prolactin levels repeated in 2 weeks.
  - The dose should be increased slowly until the prolactin level begins to decline.
  - Once prolactin levels have reliably trended down, the dose should be incrementally decreased to use the lowest dose possible while maintaining the steady improvement in prolactin levels.
  - Normalization of prolactin is not required during pregnancy, as treatment during this time is aimed at limiting growth of the mass rather than normalizing prolactin levels.
- Use of bromocriptine or cabergoline will reduce the ability of the woman to lactate after delivery.
- Surgery increases the risk of fetal loss but can be performed in the second trimester if dopamine agonist therapy fails to shrink the tumor or if vision worsens despite medication use.[3,6]
- MRI may be repeated 1–3 months after delivery to evaluate for change in tumor size.
- Cushing's disease (see Chapter 4d)
  - Treatment of Cushing's disease is necessary to reduce the risk of significant maternal and fetal complications.
  - The best treatment of Cushing's disease is transsphenoidal surgical resection.[7]

- Central hyperthyroidism
  - Treatment of central hyperthyroidism is necessary to reduce the risk of maternal and fetal complications.
  - Minimal data exist to provide optimal recommendations during pregnancy.
  - For a macroadenoma, transsphenoidal surgery to remove or reduce the tumor size is the optimal treatment and can be offered during pregnancy.
  - If surgery is not possible or if the patient opts to defer surgery until after delivery, medical management of hyperthyroidism with a β-blocker and propylthiouracil during the first trimester or methimazole during the second and third trimesters can temper the thyroidal production of thyroid hormone and symptoms of thyrotoxicosis.[8,9]
  - If surgery is not performed, regular assessment of visual fields and monitoring of compressive symptoms are essential.
- Acromegaly (see Chapter 5b)
  - Treatment of acromegaly is usually not necessary during pregnancy and can be addressed postpartum.[5]
- Nonfunctioning pituitary tumor or LH/FSH-producing pituitary tumor
  - If there is no optic nerve or chiasm involvement, treatment of a nonfunctioning pituitary tumor is usually not necessary during pregnancy but should be monitored postpartum.
- Hypopituitarism
  - Treatment of central adrenal insufficiency with glucocorticoid replacement is necessary (see Chapter 4f).
  - Treatment of central hypothyroidism with levothyroxine is necessary (see Chapter 3a).
    - For central hypothyroidism, free or total T4 levels must guide dosing of levothyroxine, as TSH is an unreliable indicator of circulating thyroid hormone levels in those with a pituitary disorder.

REFERENCES

1. Freda PU, Beckers AM, Katznelson L, et al. Pituitary incidentaloma: An endocrine society clinical practice guideline. *J Clin Endocrinol Metab.* 2011;96(4):894–904.
2. Rosmino J, Tkatch J, Di Paolo MV, Berner S, Lescano S, Guitelman M. Non-functioning pituitary adenomas and pregnancy: One-center experience and review of the literature. *Arch Endocrinol Metab.* 2021;64(5):614–622.
3. Molitch ME. Endocrinology in pregnancy: Management of the pregnant patient with a prolactinoma. *Eur J Endocrinol.* 2015;172(5):R205–R213.
4. Mastorakos G, Ilias I. Maternal and fetal hypothalamic-pituitary-adrenal axes during pregnancy and postpartum. *Ann N Y Acad Sci.* 2003;997:136–149.
5. Molitch ME. Pituitary tumors and pregnancy. *Growth Horm IGF Res.* 2003;13(Suppl A):S38–S44.
6. Brodsky JB, Cohen EN, Brown BW Jr, Wu ML, Whitcher C. Surgery during pregnancy and fetal outcome. *Am J Obstet Gynecol.* 1980;138(8):1165–1167.
7. Lindsay JR, Jonklaas J, Oldfield EH, Nieman LK. Cushing's syndrome during pregnancy: Personal experience and review of the literature. *J Clin Endocrinol Metab.* 2005;90(5):3077–3083.
8. Abuzaid H, Farouki K, Athreya A, Mahajan P. Case report: A rare case of central hyperthyroidism during pregnancy—diagnostic and therapeutic challenge. *World J Res Rev.* 2016;2(6):21–23.
9. Beck-Peccoz P, Brucker-Davis F, Persani L, Smallridge RC, Weintraub BD. Thyrotropin-secreting pituitary tumors. *Endocr Rev.* 1996;17(6):610–638.

5b

Acromegaly

MAITRI SHELLY KALIA-REYNOLDS

KEY POINTS

- Acromegaly is caused by excess growth hormone secretion from pituitary somatotroph cells and occurs most commonly in the context of a benign pituitary adenoma.
- Diagnosing acromegaly during pregnancy is challenging due to pregnancy-associated hormone fluctuations and a definitive diagnosis is typically established postpartum.
- Medical therapy for acromegaly should be discontinued during pregnancy for the majority of patients with preexisting acromegaly, as the clinical course of disease

tends to be stable, if not somewhat improved, during pregnancy.
- Medical therapy or surgery can be considered in pregnant patients with acromegaly if they have significant symptoms, including persistent headache or new visual impairment suggesting tumor growth.
- Dopamine agonists are incompatible with breastfeeding, and there is minimal data to support the use of octreotide or pegvisomant during lactation.

EPIDEMIOLOGY

- Recent studies report that acromegaly occurs with an incidence of 1.1 cases per 100,000 individuals.[1] The incidence of acromegaly in pregnant women is more uncommon due to frequent fertility impairment secondary to decreases in gonadotroph and growth hormone-releasing hormone (GHRH) that result from compressive effects of an expanding tumor mass. Simultaneous occurrence of hyperprolactinemia, as seen in mixed growth hormone (GH)-prolactin-secreting adenomas, further impairs fertility.
- More recently, pregnancy rates have somewhat risen secondary to improvements in acromegaly and fertility treatments. Most studies report that surgical, medical, and/or radiation therapy

of preexisting acromegaly increases the likelihood of successful spontaneous pregnancy and pregnancy induction.[2] There remain only limited available data on the frequency of pregnancy in uncontrolled acromegaly and in newly-diagnosed acromegaly during pregnancy.

PATHOPHYSIOLOGY

Pituitary changes in normal pregnancy

- During normal pregnancy, there is a gradual diffuse increase in maternal pituitary volume that progresses with gestational age. This is a result of increased lactotroph size and number secondary to the effect of increasing estrogen and progesterone levels.[3]

DOI: 10.1201/9781003027577-26

- The pituitary gland weight may range from 660 to 760 mg, with a corresponding volume increase of 30%.[4,5]
- Rarely, impingement on the optic chiasm and associated visual field deficits can result. These changes usually regress after delivery.
- Rising estrogen and progesterone levels are also suspected to result in relative growth hormone resistance.[6]
- The two primary isoforms of human GH include GH-normal (GH-N) and GH-variant (GH-V).
  - GH-N:
    - Secreted in a pulsatile fashion by the somatotroph cells of the anterior pituitary
    - Largely controlled by the hypothalamus through stimulatory effects of GHRH and inhibitory actions of somatostatin[6]
  - GH-V:
    - Also referred to as placental growth hormone
    - Exclusively expressed by the syncytiotrophoblasts of the placenta and is secreted into the maternal blood in a continuous fashion that is not under hypothalamic control
    - Detected as early as 8 weeks gestation[6,7]
- During the second half of a normal pregnancy, pituitary GH-N secretion substantially declines due to a negative feedback response to the progressive rise of GH-V, which becomes the predominant form of growth hormone present in maternal blood and the primary stimulus for hepatic insulin growth factor-1 (IGF-1) synthesis and secretion.[6,8]
- During the third trimester, GH-V and IGF-1 levels continue to rise to a peak around 37 weeks gestation, resulting in further suppression of GH-N.[6]

Pregnancy-related pituitary changes in acromegaly

- Acromegaly is caused by increased secretion of GH, which results in hepatic overproduction of IGF-1. The majority (95%) of acromegaly cases are attributed to a GH-secreting benign pituitary adenoma, though acromegaly can also be caused by ectopic GH production by a peripheral tumor or excessive GHRH secretion from a hypothalamic or neuroendocrine tumor.[1,9]
- Genetic syndromes that may result in acromegaly include multiple endocrine neoplasia type 1, McCune-Albright syndrome, familial acromegaly, and Carney complex.[1]
- In early pregnancy, GH resistance causes decreased IGF-1 levels via reduced production and increased turnover, potentially leading to clinical improvement of acromegaly. Unlike in normal pregnancy, in patients with acromegaly, GH-N derived from an autonomous adenoma does not respond to negative feedback from circulating GH-V or IGF-1. Therefore, after mid-gestation, concurrent elevations of GH-N and GH-V are observed.[10]
- Most patients do not experience tumor growth during pregnancy. As asymptomatic tumor growth occurred in 10% of pregnancies in one study, regular monitoring for visual field changes during pregnancy is recommended.[6,11,12]

DIAGNOSIS

- The classic physical features of acromegaly include enlarged hands and feet with broad fingers and toes. Facial deformities are often present, including a rectangular face, widened nose, prominent forehead, and enlarged lower jaw with widely spaced teeth. Patients may also present with headaches, joint and/or bone pains, fatigue, heat intolerance, or visual changes. Physical changes are typically insidious and progress slowly over years, contributing to a delay in diagnosis.[1,9,12]
- Excessive GH and IGF-1 levels also lead to adverse effects in multiple organ systems.[1,12]
  - Sleep apnea has been observed in up to 80% of patients with acromegaly due to physical obstruction associated with mandibular and maxillary growth and soft tissue thickening of the palate, tongue, and uvula.
  - Cardiac effects of acromegaly include hypertension, valvular disease, myocardial hypertrophy, or heart failure.
  - Excess GH also causes insulin resistance, with diabetes diagnosed in up to 56% of patients with acromegaly.

- Non-inflammatory, degenerative arthritis that can resemble osteoarthritis frequently occurs.
- For patients with clinical manifestations of acromegaly, the Endocrine Society guidelines recommend measuring serum IGF-1.[9] However, pregnancy complicates hormonal assessment for potential GH excess in multiple ways.
  - Frequently-used GH assays are unable to effectively differentiate pituitary GH (GH-N) from placental GH variant (GH-V), thereby leading to inaccurate results.[10]
  - As normal pregnancy is associated with reductions in GH levels and increases of IGF-1 levels, use of standard, nonpregnant reference ranges may lead to a misdiagnosis of acromegaly in pregnant patients.[6]
- Pituitary MRI is typically considered for patients presenting with symptoms of an acute intracranial process suggestive of a pituitary mass effect.[10]
- Due to the preceding challenges, a recent review suggested postponing a definitive diagnosis of acromegaly until postpartum.[6]

TREATMENT

- The treatment goals for acromegaly include normalization of GH and/or IGF-1 levels, relief of the signs and symptoms of disease, and a decrease in mortality.[13] The Endocrine Society guidelines also suggest a target biochemical goal of random GH <1.0 ng/mL and a normal age-matched IGF-1.
- For patients with acromegaly, there are three management modalities: surgery, medical therapy, and radiotherapy.
- For most patients, the primary therapy should be transsphenoidal pituitary surgery. If the disease persists post-operatively, then medications should be utilized. Medications act by either decreasing GH secretion from the pituitary, as with somatostatin receptor ligands (SRLs) and dopamine agonists, or by competitively blocking the GH receptors systemically.[9]
- SRLs include octreotide, lanreotide, and pasireotide.
  - Octreotide and lanreotide are first-generation SRLs that bind with a high affinity to somatostatin receptor (SSTR) 2 subtype. There are multiple octreotide dosage forms,

including a rapid-acting octreotide injection, long-acting release (LAR) injection, and a recently FDA-approved delayed-release oral capsule.[9,14]
  - Lanreotide is a monthly subcutaneous injection.
  - Pasireotide is a second-generation SRL that binds to both SSTR2 and SSTR5. Greater biochemical control has been demonstrated for pasireotide LAR when compared to octreotide LAR. Pasireotide LAR is associated with a higher rate of hyperglycemia and is therefore not an optimal choice for patients with poor glycemic control.[13,15]
  - For patients on long-acting SRLs, Endocrine Society guidelines recommend transitioning to short-acting octreotide two months before trying to conceive.[9] A recent review notes that patients frequently conceive while receiving long-acting SRLs and suggests measuring a human chorionic gonadotropin (hCG) level prior to each injection to minimize fetal exposure.[6]
- Dopamine agonists that may be useful for the management of acromegaly are cabergoline and bromocriptine. Dopamine agonists are less effective than SRLs and thus should be considered as medical therapy only if IGF-1 is mildly elevated (<2.5 times the upper limit of normal).[13,15] Dopamine agonists may also be added if SRL monotherapy is not providing adequate control.[15] Cabergoline is better tolerated than bromocriptine; however, there is more experience with the use of bromocriptine in pregnancy.[13,15] Dopamine agonists may result in adverse effects including gastrointestinal discomfort, hypotension, and headaches.[15]
- Pegvisomant antagonizes GH binding to its receptors and inhibits peripheral production of IGF-1. In contrast to SRLs or dopamine agonists, GH hypersecretion persists with pegvisomant therapy. Therefore, GH levels should not be monitored to evaluate for effectiveness of pegvisomant.[9] Unlike pasireotide, pegvisomant may provide the benefit of glycemic control by suppressing hepatic glucose production.[13] Liver function tests should be regularly monitored for patients receiving pegvisomant, with one study demonstrating that 5.2% of patients develop transaminase levels three times greater than normal.[15,16]

- Due to the indolent nature of acromegaly and the lack of tumor growth in the majority of patients during pregnancy, it is recommended to withhold medical therapy for acromegaly during pregnancy for the majority of patients.
  - Medical therapy may be considered if a patient develops a persistent headache or new visual impairment, potentially indicative of tumor enlargement.[6,9]
  - For patients who are intolerant to medical therapy or have symptoms of tumor growth, surgery can be considered. As general anesthesia has been associated with an increased risk of prematurity and fetal loss, transsphenoidal surgery during pregnancy is typically reserved for emergent situations. If indicated, the preferred time for surgery is the second trimester.[10,17]
- There is limited evidence to support the use of medical therapy in acromegaly for pregnant patients, as no agents have been studied in clinical trials for this population. The potential safety of medical therapy is based on animal studies and case reports.
  - Octreotide crosses the placenta and may bind to placental SSTRs.[6] In one studied patient, octreotide was associated with a short-term (less than 10 minutes) reduction in uterine artery blood flow.[18] Although low birth weight and length have been reported with octreotide use, no serious adverse fetal outcomes have been described with temporary octreotide exposure in almost 50 cases.[6,10,18]
  - The long-acting SRLs, lanreotide and pasireotide, have been associated with adverse fetal effects in animals.
  - If medical therapy is necessitated during pregnancy, dopamine agonists may be considered. There is substantial evidence supporting the safety of dopamine agonists in the management of pregnant patients with prolactinomas.[10,19,20]
  - A global database described 27 cases of maternal exposure to pegvisomant through pregnancy. Although no adverse fetal outcomes from pegvisomant were noted, many cases had incomplete data.[21]
- For patients considering breastfeeding, concurrent medical management of acromegaly is controversial as there are limited data.

- Dopamine agonists are incompatible with breastfeeding as they inhibit lactation.[22,23]
- Octreotide is excreted into breast milk; however, absorption from the oral route is unknown.[6]
- Pasireotide and lanreotide both pass into the milk of lactating rats.[24,25] Due to the potential presence in human milk and the prolonged half-life of pasireotide, it is recommended to avoid breastfeeding for 6 months after pasireotide is discontinued.[25] In a single patient, the levels of pegvisomant in the breast milk were below the lower limit of quantification of the assay.[26]

REFERENCES

1. Colao A, Grasso LFS, Giustina A, et al. Acromegaly. Nat Rev Dis Primers. Mar 21, 2019; 5(1):20.
2. Grynberg M, Salenave S, Young J, et al. Female gonadal function before and after treatment of acromegaly. J of Clin Endocrinol Metab. Oct 2010; 95(10):4518–25.
3. Pivonello R, De Martino MC, Auriemma RS, et al. Pituitary tumors and pregnancy: The interplay between a pathologic condition and a physiologic status. J Endocrinol Invest. Feb 2014; 37(2):99–112.
4. Gonzalez JG, Elizondo G, Saldivar D, et al. Pituitary gland growth during normal pregnancy: An in vivo study using magnetic resonance imaging. Am J Med. Aug 1988; 85(2):217–20.
5. Dinç J, Esen F, Demirci A, et al. Pituitary dimensions and volume measurements in pregnancy and postpartum. MR assessment. Acta Radiol. Jan 1998; 39(1):64–9.
6. Abucham J, Bronstein MD, Dias ML. Management of endocrine disease: Acromegaly and pregnancy: A contemporary review. Eur J Endocrinol. Jul 2017; 177(1):R1–R12.
7. Muhammad A, Neggers SJ, van der Lely AJ. Pregnancy and acromegaly. Pituitary. Feb 2017; 20(1):179–184.
8. Newbern D, Freemark M. Placental hormones and the control of maternal metabolism and fetal growth. Curr Opin Endocrinol Diabetes Obes. Dec 2011; 18(6):409–16.

9. Katznelson L, Laws Jr ER, Melmed S, et al. Acromegaly: An Endocrine Society clinical practice guideline. J Clin Endocrinol Metab. Nov 2014; 99(11):3933–51.

10. Huang W, Molitch ME. Pituitary tumors in pregnancy. Endocrinol Metab Clin North Am. Sep 2019; 48(3):569–81.

11. Caron P, Broussaud S, Bertherat, J, et al. Acromegaly and pregnancy: A retrospective multicenter study of 59 pregnancies in 46 women. J Clin Endocrinol Metab. Oct 2010; 95(10):4680–7.

12. Katznelson L, Atkinson JK, Cook DM, et al. American Association of Clinical Endocrinologists medical guidelines for clinical practice for the diagnosis and treatment of acromegaly—2011 update. Endocr Pract. Jul–Aug 2011; 17(Suppl 4):1–44.

13. Melmed S, Bronstein MD, Chanson P, et al. A consensus statement on acromegaly therapeutic outcomes. Nat Rev Endocrinol. Sep 2018; 14(9):552–61.

14. Octreotide. Mycapssa delayed-release capsules package insert. Chiasma. Revised 6/2020.

15. Shanik MH. Limitations of current approaches for the treatment of acromegaly. Endocr Pract. Feb 2016; 22(2):210–9.

16. Schreiber I, Buchfelder M, Droste M, et al. Treatment of acromegaly with the GH receptor antagonist pegvisomant in clinical practice: Safety and efficacy evaluation from the German pegvisomant observational study. Eur J Endocrinol. Jan 2007; 156(1):75–82.

17. Cheng V, Faiman C, Kennedy L, et al. Pregnancy and acromegaly: A review. Pituitary. Mar 2012; 15(1):59–63.

18. Maffei P, Tamagno G, Nardelli GB, et al. Effects of octreotide exposure during pregnancy in acromegaly. Clin Endocrin (Oxf). 2010; 72:668–77.

19. Woodmansee WW. Pituitary disorders in pregnancy. Neurol Clin. Feb 2019; 37(1):63–83.

20. Molitch ME. Prolactinoma in pregnancy. Best Pract Res Clin Endocrinol Metab. 2011; 25:885–96.

21. van der Lely AJ, Gomez R, Heissler JF, et al. Pregnancy in acromegaly patients treated with pegvisomant. Endocrine. Aug 2015; 49(3):769–73.

22. Rains CP, Bryson HM, Fitton A. Cabergoline. A review of its pharmacological properties and therapeutic potential in the treatment of hyperprolactinaemia and inhibition of lactation. Drugs. Feb 1995; 49(2):255–79.

23. Assal A, Malcom J, Lochnan H, et al. Preconception counselling for women with acromegaly: More questions than answers. Obstet Med. Mar 2016; 9(1):9–14.

24. Lanreotide. Somatuline depot injection package insert. Ipsen. Revised 6/2019.

25. Pasireotide. Signifor package insert. Novartis. Revised 1/2020.

26. Brian Sr, Bidlingmaier M, Wajnrajch MP, et al. Treatment of acromegaly with pegvisomant during pregnancy: Maternal and fetal effects. J Clin Endocrinol Metab. Sep 2007; 92(9):3374–77.

5c

Growth hormone deficiency

BEATRIZ FRANCESCA RAMIREZ

KEY POINTS

- The data on incidence and prevalence of growth hormone deficiency (GHD) in children and adults is limited.
- In the first trimester of pregnancy, pituitary growth hormone (GH-N) is the predominant form of growth hormone (GH) in the maternal serum. During the second and third trimesters, placental GH (GH-V) is the main regulator of insulin-like growth factor-1 (IGF-1) levels in pregnancy. As GH-V levels rise, GH secretion by pituitary somatotrophs is inhibited.
- During pregnancy, diagnosis of GHD is challenging because interference of circulating placental hormones homologous to GH-N can often lead to either falsely elevated or suppressed values in GH assays.
- GH-V levels in patients with GHD are not different from GH-V levels in normal subjects. During the third trimester, IGF-1 concentrations rise to a similar degree during pregnancy in patients with or without GHD.
- Several studies support treatment of women with recombinant human GH (rhGH) while seeking fertility. Continuing rhGH during pregnancy does not appear to impact the outcome for either mother or fetus; therefore, it is often discontinued during pregnancy.

EPIDEMIOLOGY

- GHD in adults can be categorized into three main groups[1]:
  - Childhood-onset
    - Can be further divided into organic and idiopathic causes
  - Acquired (lesions or trauma)
  - Idiopathic
- In adults, the causes of GHD are the same as the causes of deficiencies of other pituitary hormones or hypopituitarism. A study of adults with hypopituitarism in which acromegaly and Cushing's disease were excluded demonstrated the following etiologies[2]:

- Pituitary tumor or consequences of treatment including surgery and radiation (76%)
- Extra-pituitary tumor (craniopharyngioma, metastatic disease) (13%)
- Unknown cause (8%)
- Sarcoidosis (1%)
- Sheehan syndrome (0.5%)
- The data on incidence and prevalence of GHD in children and adults is limited, with findings of 1.2–33 per 100,000 per year to 4.6–40.6 per 100,000 per year, respectively. The reason for this variability may be related to the lack of a standardized approach to diagnosis of hypopituitarism or GHD, which impedes epidemiologic assessment.[3]

DOI: 10.1201/9781003027577-27

119

- The incidence and prevalence of GHD are higher in males compared to females.
- The prevalence of isolated GHD in children is estimated at 1 per 4,000 to 1 per 10,000.[4]
- In pregnant women, there is no current data on the incidence and prevalence of GHD.

PATHOPHYSIOLOGY

Somatotropic axis during normal pregnancy

- Embryo implantation and trophoblast growth result in development of the placenta. The placenta functions to coordinate the maternal hormonal environment to ensure the growth of the fetus.[5]
- The placenta produces placental growth hormone (GH-V) and human placental lactogen (hPL). Both of these are responsible for stimulation of IGF-1, which increases insulin resistance in the mother, thereby directing glucose to the fetus and promoting fetal growth.[6]
- In the first trimester, GH-N is the predominant form of GH in the maternal serum. It does not cross the placenta and is not necessary for gestation and normal fetal development, as has been demonstrated in pregnancies in GH-deficient patients.
- During this period, rising estradiol levels induce a state of GH resistance as reflected by a significant decline in IGF-1 levels. After this, GH-V levels begin to rise and overcome GH resistance as reflected by increasing IGF-1 levels.[7]
- GH-V binds with the same affinity as GH-N to the GH receptor (GHR) and does not cross the placenta.
- During the second and third trimesters, GH-V is the main regulator of IGF-1 levels and its concentration is higher than GH-N starting from week 20 of gestation. A progressive rise in GH-V is associated with a constant decline in the secretion of GH-N. At gestational week 36, the GH-V level is comparable to GH levels in women with acromegaly.
- In summary, the placenta regulates the somatotropic system during pregnancy, as it becomes the main source of GH, while GH secretion by pituitary somatotrophs is inhibited.[5]

Effect of GHD on the gonadotropic axis

- GH and IGF-1 regulate the hypothalamic-pituitary-gonadal axis throughout life, beginning with the regulation of puberty onset. GH influences the release of gonadotropins from the pituitary, estradiol production by granulosa cells, oocyte maturation, fertility, and lactation. GH also enhances the ovarian response to gonadotropins.[7]
- The IGF system is one of the main intraovarian regulators of follicular development and sex steroid production. In the ovary, IGF-1 and IGF-2 receptors are expressed. IGF-1 stimulates proliferation and activity of granulosa cells. The IGF system in the ovaries receives information from insulin and GH signaling pathways and contributes to the control of ovarian functions such as initiation of puberty and ovulation.[5]
- Animal experiments have demonstrated that disturbances in GH signaling affect embryonic and placental development and that the rise in maternal IGF-1 during early pregnancy is important for the normal morphology and function of the placenta. In GHR knockout mice, fetal size and pup weight are significantly lower.[5]
- In women, GHD has been associated with delayed onset of puberty, smaller uterine size, amenorrhea in 60% of cases, and polycystic ovarian morphology in 75% of cases.
- Patients with Laron syndrome (a condition caused by a genetic abnormality of the GHR in which there is complete insensitivity to GH) have smaller gonads and genitalia as well as delayed onset of puberty.[8,9] The role of GH at conception is not clear given that normal ovulation and fertility can be observed in individuals with Laron syndrome and other causes of GH resistance.[8]

DIAGNOSIS

- Pregnant women can present with either childhood or adult-onset GHD. In both situations, the diagnosis of GHD is usually already established with no need for further diagnostic testing during pregnancy. As pregnancy advances, GH-V dominates control of IGF-1 secretion, leading to challenges in diagnosing GHD during pregnancy.

- Interference of circulating placental hormones with homology to GH-N can often lead to falsely elevated or suppressed GH values in GH assays.[10]
- Serum IGF-1 levels are elevated in normal pregnancy toward mid-gestation and onward, which also complicates diagnosis of GHD.[5,7]
- Provocative testing to diagnose GHD in pregnant women may be unsafe to perform during gestation and is not encountered in medical literature. Thus, evaluation for GHD should be delayed until after delivery.
- If a pregnant woman presents with GHD acquired in adulthood, other pituitary hormonal deficiencies should be suspected and the patient should be evaluated and treated if not done previously.

TREATMENT

- Several studies confirmed that GH replacement improves amenorrhea/dysmenorrhea and may improve fertility in patients with GHD. This includes problems with ovulation in women with GHD that improve after implementation of GH replacement therapy (GHRT) with resultant spontaneous conceptions.[5,11]
- In pregnancy, deficiency of GH-N does not appear to affect placental secretion of GH or IGF-1. Therefore, it is questionable whether there is a role for GHRT during pregnancy.
- There is clinical evidence that women with childhood-onset GHD have worse pregnancy outcomes than women with adult-onset GHD.[5]

Controversies of treatment with rhGH during pregnancy

- GHRT during conception and pregnancy has not been endorsed by any of the major endocrine organizations. However, data from clinical care practice shows that most women conceive while on GHRT and studies have shown more than half of women continue GHRT during pregnancy.[5]
- The American Association of Clinical Endocrinology (AACE) Growth Hormone Task Force in 2019 recognized that several studies support the use of rhGH while seeking fertility, and continuing rhGH during pregnancy does not appear to impact the outcome for either mother or fetus. It was concluded that more data is needed and routine use of rhGH during conception or pregnancy cannot be recommended at this time.[12]
- The KIMS study in Vienna, which assessed pregnancies in a large group of patients with GHD and hypopituitarism concluded that there is no relation between GHRT regimens and pregnancy outcomes.[11]
- If treatment of GHD during pregnancy is continued, it is difficult to adjust rhGH dose based on serum IGF-1 during pregnancy and, in general, prepregnancy doses are continued during the first trimester.[5,13] GHRT is often discontinued after the first trimester.
- Unwanted side effects of GHRT may be exacerbated in pregnancy, including peripheral edema, arthralgias, carpal tunnel syndrome, paresthesias, and worsening glucose tolerance.[5,14] Very rarely, macular edema has been described.
- Active malignancy is a contraindication to treatment with rhGH.
- GH and lactation
  - Experiments in rats have shown the complementary effects of GH and prolactin on the synthesis and secretion of breast milk. GH appears to maintain the synthesis and secretion of high fat, energy-dense breast milk, an effect elicited by the action of GH directly on the mammary gland. Prolactin has major effects on mammary tissues and breast milk synthesis.[15]
  - In humans, studies of mothers with lactational insufficiency have shown that GHRT can improve breast milk volume without adverse effects on mothers or their infants.[16,17] Recombinant hGH treatment did not appear to affect breast milk constituents, and levels of rhGH and IGF-1 in breast milk remained low regardless of rhGH dose.[18]

REFERENCES

1. Molitch ME, Clemmons DR, Malozowski S, Merriam GR, Shalet SM, Vance ML; Endocrine Society's Clinical Guidelines Subcommittee, Stephens PA. Evaluation

and treatment of adult growth hormone deficiency: an Endocrine Society Clinical Practice Guideline. J Clin Endocrinol Metab. 2006 May;91(5):1621–34.

2. Bates AS, Van't Hoff W, Jones PJ, Clayton RN. The effect of hypopituitarism on life expectancy. J Clin Endocrinol Metab. 1996 Mar;81(3):1169–72.

3. Stochholm K, Christiansen JS. The Epidemiology of Growth Hormone Deficiency [Internet]. SpringerLink. Humana Press; 1970 [cited 2020Sep11]. Available from: https://link.springer.com/chapter/10.1007/978-1-60761-317-6_8

4. Stanley T. Diagnosis of growth hormone deficiency in childhood. Curr Opin Endocrinol Diabetes Obes. 2012 Feb;19(1):47–52.

5. Vila G, Luger A. Growth hormone deficiency and pregnancy: any role for substitution? Minerva Endocrinol. 2018 Dec;43(4):451–57.

6. Alsat E, Guibourdenche J, Couturier A, Evain-Brion D. Physiological role of human placental growth hormone. Mol Cell Endocrinol. 1998 May 25;140(1–2):121–27.

7. Abucham J, Bronstein MD, Dias ML. Management of endocrine disease: acromegaly and pregnancy: a contemporary review. Eur J Endocrinol. 2017 Jul;177(1):R1–12.

8. Laron Z. Prismatic cases: Laron syndrome (primary growth hormone resistance) from patient to laboratory to patient. J Clin Endocrinol Metab. 1995 May;80(5):1526–31.

9. Latrech H, Polak M. Syndrome de Laron: aspects diagnostiques, thérapeutiques et pronostiques [Laron syndrome: Presentation, treatment and prognosis]. Presse Med. 2016 Jan;45(1):40–45. French.

10. Obuobie K, Mullik V, Jones C, John R, Rees AE, Davies JS, Scanlon MF, Lazarus JH. McCune-Albright syndrome: growth hormone dynamics in pregnancy. J Clin Endocrinol Metab. 2001 Jun;86(6):2456–58.

11. Vila G, Akerblad AC, Mattsson AF, Riedl M, Webb SM, Hána V, Nielsen EH, Biller BM, Luger A. Pregnancy outcomes in women with growth hormone deficiency. Fertil Steril. 2015 Nov;104(5):1210–7.e1.

12. Yuen KCJ, Biller BMK, Radovick S, Carmichael JD, Jasim S, Pantalone KM, Hoffman AR. American association of clinical endocrinologists and American College of Endocrinology guidelines for management of growth hormone deficiency in adults and patients transitioning from pediatric to adult care. Endocr Pract. 2019 Nov;25(11):1191–1232.

13. Møller N, Jørgensen JO. Effects of growth hormone on glucose, lipid, and protein metabolism in human subjects. Endocr Rev. 2009 Apr;30(2):152–77.

14. Holmes SJ, Shalet SM. Which adults develop side-effects of growth hormone replacement? Clin Endocrinol (Oxf). 1995 Aug;43(2):143–49.

15. Flint DJ, Gardner M. Evidence that growth hormone stimulates milk synthesis by direct action on the mammary gland and that prolactin exerts effects on milk secretion by maintenance of mammary deoxyribonucleic acid content and tight junction status. Endocrinology. 1994 Sep;135(3):1119–24.

16. Gunn AJ, Gunn TR, Rabone DL, Breier BH, Blum WF, Gluckman PD. Growth hormone increases breast milk volumes in mothers of preterm infants. Pediatrics. 1996 Aug;98(2 Pt 1):279–82.

17. Milsom SR, Rabone DL, Gunn AJ, Gluckman PD. Potential role for growth hormone in human lactation insufficiency. Horm Res. 1998 Sep;50(3):147–50.

18. Milsom SR, Breier BH, Gallaher BW, Cox VA, Gunn AJ, Gluckman PD. Growth hormone stimulates galactopoiesis in healthy lactating women. Acta Endocrinol (Copenh). 1992 Oct;127(4):337–43.

Hyperprolactinemia

KRYSTEL FEGHALI AND GAYATRI JAISWAL

KEY POINTS

- Prolactin levels and pituitary gland size normally increase throughout pregnancy. Therefore, it is not recommended to monitor prolactin levels during pregnancy.
- In pregnant women with known prolactinomas, visual symptoms should be monitored and evaluated with formal visual field testing if any vision changes are noted.
- For patients previously on dopamine agonists with stable tumor size on MRI prior to conception, it is generally recommended that dopamine agonist therapy be discontinued upon confirmation of pregnancy.
- Dopamine agonists are recommended as first-line therapy for prolactinoma growth during pregnancy. For adenomas with lack of response with worsening visual symptoms, transsphenoidal surgery can be performed in the second trimester.

EPIDEMIOLOGY

- Prolactinomas are adenomas that arise from lactotroph cells in the pituitary gland which secrete prolactin. They are the most common type of functioning pituitary tumor and account for 40% of all pituitary adenomas.[1]
- Prolactinomas occur with a prevalence of 60–100 cases per million. Occurrence is more common in women. The highest incidence rate was 23.9/100,000 person-years and most common in women between 25 and 34 years of age.
- In women, prolactinomas are more commonly microadenomas measuring less than 1 cm.[1]
- Microprolactinomas tend to follow a benign course throughout pregnancy. Asymptomatic growth occurs in 4.5% of the cases, whereas symptomatic growth occurs in <2%.[1]
- Macroprolactinomas undergo symptomatic growth in 20–30% of patients during pregnancy. The risk increases with increasing tumor size and extrasellar extension.[1]
- Current literature suggests that pregnancy induces remission of hyperprolactinemia in two-thirds of patients after discontinuation of dopamine agonists, likely mediated by tumor auto-infarction. Remission rates[1]:
  - 76–100% of nontumoral (idiopathic) hyperprolactinemia
  - 66–70% in microprolactinomas
  - 64–70% in macroprolactinomas

PATHOPHYSIOLOGY

- Lactotroph cells located in the anterior pituitary secrete prolactin, which serves as an essential mediator of breast milk production and lactation.
- Dopamine inhibits growth of lactotrophs and secretion of prolactin.[2]

DOI: 10.1201/9781003027577-28

- Prolactin levels and pituitary gland size increase throughout pregnancy. This is mediated by lactotroph cell hyperplasia secondary to the increased estrogenic stimulatory effect on pituitary lactotrophs.[1]
- Prolactinoma size can also increase in response to the estrogen elevation in pregnancy.[2]
- During pregnancy, prolactin levels rise as high as 400 ng/mL.[3] This prolactin elevation prepares the mammary glands for lactation.[4]
- Microprolactinomas rarely increase in size during pregnancy and patients commonly remain asymptomatic.
- Macroprolactinomas increase in size in approximately one-third of patients during pregnancy and can be associated with headaches and an increased risk of optic nerve and chiasm compression with visual field symptoms.

DIAGNOSIS

- The majority of prolactinomas in pregnant patients are diagnosed prior to conception.
- During pregnancy, prolactin levels may not rise with tumor enlargement.[5] In addition, prolactin levels are expected to be high in a normal pregnancy. For these reasons, prolactin levels may be misleading, therefore serum prolactin measurement during pregnancy is not recommended.
- Some experts suggest that prolactin measurement during pregnancy in patients with prolactinomas can be reassuring if levels remain <400 ng/mL. When levels rise >400 ng/mL, visual field testing may be obtained.
- Visual field testing
  - During pregnancy, routine visual field testing is not recommended.
  - Visual field testing should be obtained for women who develop visual symptoms.
  - For women with pituitary macroadenomas extending above the sella, it is recommended that visual field testing be performed before pregnancy and every three months during pregnancy regardless of visual symptoms.
- Imaging
  - Pituitary MRI is recommended prior to conception to document tumor size and serve as a baseline. Thereafter, routine MRI is not indicated during pregnancy.
  - MRI without gadolinium is recommended in pregnant women who experience headaches and/or visual field abnormalities (bitemporal hemianopsia) to assess adenoma size.

TREATMENT

- Pregnant patients with prolactinomas should be counseled regarding the natural history of the prolactinoma prior to conception with a clear plan for monitoring throughout pregnancy.[4]
- Tumor growth is dependent on the adenoma size prior to pregnancy (3–4.5% for microadenomas versus 20–32% for macroadenomas).[1,6] Women with prolactinomas, and particularly macroadenomas, should be monitored closely during pregnancy.
- Pregnant patients should be seen at routine intervals and followed for development of new or worsening headaches and/or changes in vision[4]:
  - Microadenomas: Follow-up recommended every three months.
  - Macroadenomas: Follow-up recommended at least every three months and more frequently with larger adenomas.
- If treatment is necessary due to significant adenoma growth with visual impairment, dopamine agonists are first-line therapy for prolactinomas.[2] Up to 90% of prolactinomas are responsive to cabergoline and 70–80% of prolactinomas are responsive to bromocriptine.[7]
- Bromocriptine has the largest safety database and has a proven safety record for pregnancy. The data regarding use of cabergoline in pregnancy is smaller; however, to date, there is no evidence indicating that it exerts deleterious effects on the developing fetus.[2]
- To limit exposure time of the developing fetus to dopamine agonists, therapy is recommended for the shortest duration possible during pregnancy. Discontinuation of the drug at confirmation of pregnancy is usually recommended. When discontinued early, dopamine agonists have not been found to increase the risk of spontaneous abortions, ectopic pregnancies, trophoblastic disease, multiple pregnancies, or congenital malformations.[8]

- If the patient was previously on dopamine agonist therapy prior to pregnancy, use of the same dopamine agonist previously tolerated is recommended.
- If bromocriptine was initially used without adenoma response, cabergoline should then be initiated.[9]
- If pharmacologic therapy is not successful in alleviating visual symptoms, transsphenoidal surgery in the second trimester is recommended. In the third trimester, surgery for persistent symptoms should be deferred until after delivery, if possible.[1]
- A minority of patients with microadenomas or intrasellar macroadenomas may choose transsphenoidal surgery. In contrast to medical management, transsphenoidal surgery results in permanent normalization of prolactin levels in only 60% of cases and is associated with some morbidity and mortality.[2]
- Breastfeeding considerations
  - Dopamine agonists impair prolactin secretion and hence lactation.
  - Patients should be counseled on possible inability to breastfeed after use of dopamine agonist therapy during pregnancy.
  - For women who required dopamine agonist therapy throughout pregnancy and who wish to breastfeed, an MRI should be performed postpartum prior to discontinuation of dopamine agonist therapy to ensure stability of the adenoma and detect asymptomatic tumor growth.[1]
  - Dopamine agonists can then be resumed following cessation of lactation if needed.

REFERENCES

1. Almalki MH, Alzahrani S, Alshahrani F, Alsherbeni S, Almoharib O, Aljohani N, et al. Managing Prolactinomas during Pregnancy. *Front Endocrinol (Lausanne)*. 2015;6:85.
2. Molitch ME. Endocrinology in Pregnancy: Management of the Pregnant Patient with a Prolactinoma. *Eur J Endocrinol*. 2015;172(5):R205–R213.
3. Bronstein MD. Prolactinomas and Pregnancy. *Pituitary*. 2005;8(1):31–38.
4. Melmed S, Casanueva FF, Hoffman AR, et al. Diagnosis and Treatment of Hyperprolactinemia: an Endocrine Society Clinical Practice Guideline. *J Clin Endocrinol Metab*. 2011;96(2):273–288.
5. Divers WA Jr, Yen SS. Prolactin-Producing Microadenomas in Pregnancy. *Obstet Gynecol*. 1983;62(4):425–429.
6. Gillam MP, Molitch ME, Lombardi G, Colao A. Advances in the Treatment of Prolactinomas. *Endocr Rev*. 2006;27(5):485–534.
7. Maiter D. Management of Dopamine Agonist-Resistant Prolactinoma. *Neuroendocrinology*. 2019;109(1):42–50.
8. Molitch ME. Prolactinoma in Pregnancy. *Best Pract Res Clin Endocrinol Metab*. 2011;25(6):885–896.
9. Liu C, Tyrrell JB. Successful Treatment of a Large Macroprolactinoma with Cabergoline during Pregnancy. *Pituitary*. 2001;4(3):179–185.

Nonfunctioning sellar masses

OKSANA SYMCZYK

KEY POINTS

- Craniopharyngiomas are rare benign tumors that arise from remnant epithelial cells of Rathke's pouch.
- Rathke cleft cysts are comprised of epithelium-lined intrasellar cysts located between the anterior and posterior lobes of the pituitary gland.
- Rathke cleft cysts are typically small and discovered incidentally on imaging.
- Craniopharyngiomas and Rathke cleft cysts in pregnancy can present with clinical symptoms

including headache and visual disturbances in addition to hormone abnormalities including panhypopituitarism and/or diabetes insipidus.
- The recommended treatment of craniopharyngiomas with optic nerve compression or hypopituitarism is transsphenoidal surgical resection.
- Rathke cleft cysts usually do not require treatment during pregnancy unless large and associated with compressive symptoms and/or pituitary hormone dysfunction.

CRANIOPHARYNGIOMA

Epidemiology

- Craniopharyngiomas are rare in the general population, comprising 1–3% of all brain tumors.[1]
- Craniopharyngiomas account for 5–10% of brain tumors among patients up to 19 years of age.[1,2]
- Only nine documented cases have been reported in pregnancy with one case describing disease recurrence.
- With treatment, overall survival rates at 3 years are greater than 85%.[2]

Pathophysiology

- Craniopharyngiomas are circumscribed epithelial tumors arising in the suprasellar region.
- Craniopharyngiomas are typically benign. Due to the tumor's location, however, pituitary

gland compression and hormone dysfunction are common. In addition, these tumors can lead to compression of the optic chiasm which is located superiorly to the pituitary gland, resulting in visual defects.
- There are two clinically distinct subtypes[2,3]:
  - Adamantinomatous
    - Most common type of craniopharyngioma
    - Arises from mutations in the beta-catenin gene
  - Papillary
    - Occurs almost exclusively in adults
    - Arises from BRAF gene mutations

Diagnosis

- Symptoms
  - A combination of headache, visual impairment, polydipsia and polyuria, and/or signs

DOI: 10.1201/9781003027577-29

of anterior pituitary hormonal deficiencies should raise suspicion.

- Most symptoms are related to increased intracranial pressure.
- Tumors may increase in size during pregnancy and lead to compression of the optic chiasm, resulting in[4,5]:
  - Visual field defects
  - Papilledema
  - Optic atrophy
- Compression of the pituitary commonly results in anterior and posterior pituitary dysfunction, with symptoms of adrenal insufficiency, hypothyroidism, hypogonadism, and diabetes insipidus.[6,7]
- A sudden-onset, severe headache associated with visual impairment and hypotension suggests pituitary apoplexy, a bleed into the pituitary which is considered a medical emergency requiring immediate treatment with glucocorticoids and neurosurgical consultation (see Chapter 5i).[8]
- Biochemical testing may reveal deficiencies in any or all of the following hormones:
  - Insulin-like growth factor 1 (IGF-1) as a measure of growth hormone
  - Thyroid-stimulating hormone (TSH) with concomitant free thyroxine (T4)
  - 8 AM plasma or serum cortisol
  - Prolactin
- Imaging
  - Magnetic resonance imaging (MRI) with gadolinium is the diagnostic test of choice for most sellar masses, however, gadolinium is contraindicated in pregnancy. MRI without gadolinium performed in the second or third trimester may aid in the diagnosis.[9-19]
  - Imaging appearance
    - Adamantinomatous craniopharyngiomas are typically lobulated, cystic, and usually associated with calcifications. They often demonstrate local invasion.
    - Papillary craniopharyngiomas are well-circumscribed and predominantly solid tumors or mixed solid-cystic spherical tumors in the suprasellar region. This subtype typically develops in the third ventricle.
  - Head CT can be useful in detecting tumor calcifications (a common finding in craniopharyngiomas) but is not advised in pregnancy.

Treatment

- Formal visual field examination is recommended for pregnant patients noting visual disturbances.
- Surgery is the recommended treatment for craniopharyngiomas. The goal of treatment is to achieve complete resection of all tumor cells.
- Although craniopharyngiomas are benign tumors, if not completely resected they have the potential to recur locally.
- Approximately 50% of patients require multiple surgeries to control tumor growth.[20]
- Surgical approach is chosen based upon the location and size of the tumor as well as its relationship to other structures such as the pituitary gland, infundibulum, diaphragma sellae, third ventricle and optic chiasm.
- In pregnant patients, transsphenoidal approach is the safest surgical option when the tumor is localized to the intrasellar region. If complete tumor resection is not possible with a transsphenoidal approach, transcranial resection can be considered in the postpartum period.
- The most common complication following either type of surgery is central diabetes insipidus which occurs in 90% of patients and remains permanent in 60–80% of patients.[21]
- In pregnant patients whose tumors are felt to be inoperable or in whom risks of surgical resection are not acceptable, radiation in the postpartum period may also be considered.

RATHKE CLEFT CYST

Epidemiology

- Rathke cleft cysts have been reported as incidental findings in 4–33% of autopsy cases.[22]
- There is a female to male ratio of 3:1.
- Usually diagnosed between 30 and 50 years of age

Pathophysiology

- Rathke cleft cysts are benign, congenital lesions of the sella.

- They originate from embryonic remnants of Rathke's pouch which appears on the 24th day of embryonic life:
  - The craniopharyngeal duct forms as Rathke's pouch extends cranially; meanwhile, the infundibulum forms from the diencephalon as a downgrowth of the neuroepithelium.
  - Between the third and fifth month of gestation, cells in the anterior wall of Rathke's pouch proliferate to form the anterior pituitary.
  - The infundibulum differentiates into the median eminence, the pituitary stalk, and the posterior pituitary lobe.
  - Failure of obliteration of the craniopharyngeal duct results in the development of a cyst between the pars distalis of the anterior pituitary and the pars nervosa of the posterior pituitary.[23]

Diagnosis

- Symptoms
  - A combination of headache, visual impairment, polydipsia and polyuria, and/or signs of anterior pituitary hormonal deficiencies should raise suspicion.[24]
  - Most symptoms are related to increased intracranial pressure.
  - Tumors may increase in size during pregnancy and lead to compression of the optic chiasm, resulting in[4,5]:
    - Visual field defects
    - Papilledema
    - Optic atrophy
  - Compression of the pituitary commonly results in anterior and posterior pituitary dysfunction, with symptoms of adrenal insufficiency, hypothyroidism, hypogonadism, and diabetes insipidus.[6,7]
  - While pituitary apoplexy is rare with Rathke cleft cysts, some case reports have been described. If apoplexy is diagnosed, immediate glucocorticoid administration and neurosurgical consultation is indicated.[24,25]
- Biochemical testing may reveal deficiencies in any or all of the following hormones:
  - Insulin-like growth factor 1 (IGF-1) as a measure of growth hormone

- Thyroid-stimulating hormone (TSH) with concomitant free thyroxine (T4)
- 8 AM plasma or serum cortisol
- Prolactin
- Imaging:
  - Magnetic resonance imaging (MRI) with gadolinium is the diagnostic test of choice for most sellar masses, however gadolinium is contraindicated in pregnancy. MRI without gadolinium performed in the second or third trimester may aid in the diagnosis.[10–19,23]
  - Imaging appearance:
    - Well-circumscribed, spherical, or ovoid lesions in the central sellar region
    - Cystic lesions with smooth contours and without calcification or rim enhancement
    - Usually <3 mm in size
    - May increase in volume during pregnancy, but typically remain stable
- Definitive diagnosis:
  - Cyst wall biopsy, although not typically performed during pregnancy

Treatment

- Formal visual field examination is recommended for pregnant patients noting visual disturbances.
- Treatment of Rathke cleft cysts is symptom-dependent:
  - Small Rathke cleft cysts that do not cause any symptoms do not require treatment.
  - For those presenting solely with headache, conservative symptom management is recommended.[26]
  - Larger, symptomatic Rathke cleft cysts may require surgery, including drainage and cyst resection typically via a transsphenoidal approach, preferably in the second trimester.

REFERENCES

1. Bunin GR, Surawicz TS, Witman PA, Preston-Martin S, Davis F, Bruner JM. The descriptive epidemiology of craniopharyngioma. J Neurosurg. 1998;89(4):547–51.
2. Zacharia BE, Bruce SS, Goldstein H, Malone HR, Neugut AI, Bruce JN. Incidence,

treatment and survival of patients with craniopharyngioma in the surveillance, epidemiology and end results program. *Neuro Oncol.* 2012;14(8):1070–78.

3. Müller HL, Merchant TE, Warmuth-Metz M, Martinez-Barbera JP, Puget S. Craniopharyngioma. *Nat Rev Dis Primers.* 2019;5(1):75.

4. Aydin Y, Can SM, Gülkilik A, Türkmenoglu O, Alatli C, Ziyal I. Rapid enlargement and recurrence of a preexisting intrasellar craniopharyngioma during the course of two pregnancies. Case report. *J Neurosurg.* 1999;91(2):322–24.

5. Maniker AH, Krieger AJ. Rapid recurrence of craniopharyngioma during pregnancy with recovery of vision: A case report. *Surg Neurol.* 1996;45(4):324–27.

6. van der Wildt B, Drayer JI, Eskes TK. Diabetes insipidus in pregnancy as a first sign of a craniopharyngioma. *Eur J Obstet Gynecol Reprod Biol.* 1980;10(4):269–74.

7. Hiett AK, Barton JR. Diabetes insipidus associated with craniopharyngioma in pregnancy. *Int J Gynaecol Obstet.* 1991;35(4):378–78.

8. Zoia C, Cattalani A, Turpini E, Custodi VM, Benazzo M, Pagella F, et al. Haemorrhagic presentation of a craniopharyngioma in a pregnant woman. *Case Rep Neurol Med.* 2014;2014:435208.

9. Jain C. ACOG committee opinion no. 723: Guidelines for diagnostic imaging during pregnancy and lactation. *Obstet Gynecol.* 2019;133(1):186.

10. Acr.org. [cited 2021 Apr 9]. Available from: https://www.acr.org/-/media/ACR/Files/Radiology-Safety/MR-Safety/Manual-on-MR-Safety.pdf

11. Amin R, Darrah T, Wang H, Amin S. Editor's highlight: In utero exposure to gadolinium and adverse neonatal outcomes in premature infants. *Toxicol Sci.* 2017;156(2):520–26.

12. Bird ST, Gelperin K, Sahin L, Bleich KB, Fazio-Eynullayeva E, Woods C, et al. First-trimester exposure to gadolinium-based contrast agents: A utilization study of 4.6 million U.S. pregnancies. *Radiology.* 2019;293(1):193–200.

13. Chartier AL, Bouvier MJ, McPherson DR, Stepenosky JE, Taysom DA, Marks RM. The safety of maternal and fetal MRI at 3 T. *AJR Am J Roentgenol.* 2019;213(5):1170–73.

14. Kallmes DF, Watson RE Jr. Gadolinium administration in undetected pregnancy: Cause for alarm? *Radiology.* 2019;293(1):201–2.

15. Mervak BM, Altun E, McGinty KA, Hyslop WB, Semelka RC, Burke LM. MRI in pregnancy: Indications and practical considerations: MRI in pregnancy. *J Magn Reson Imaging.* 2019;49(3):621–31.

16. Murata N, Gonzalez-Cuyar LF, Murata K, Fligner C, Dills R, Hippe D, et al. Macrocyclic and other non-Group 1 gadolinium contrast agents deposit low levels of gadolinium in brain and bone tissue: Preliminary results from 9 patients with normal renal function. *Invest Radiol.* 2016;51(7):447–53.

17. Patenaude Y, Pugash D, Lim K, Morin L, Lim K, Bly S, et al. The use of magnetic resonance imaging in the obstetric patient. *J Obstet Gynaecol Can.* 2014;36(4):349–55.

18. Ray JG, Vermeulen MJ, Bharatha A, Montanera WJ, Park AL. Association between MRI exposure during pregnancy and fetal and childhood outcomes. *JAMA.* 2016;316(9):952.

19. Rogosnitzky M, Branch S. Gadolinium-based contrast agent toxicity: A review of known and proposed mechanisms. *Biometals.* 2016;29(3):365–76.

20. Mortini P, Losa M, Pozzobon G, Barzaghi R, Riva M, Acerno S, et al. Neurosurgical treatment of craniopharyngioma in adults and children: Early and long-term results in a large case series: Clinical article. *J Neurosurg.* 2011;114(5):1350–59.

21. Gleeson H, Amin R, Maghnie M. "Do no harm": Management of craniopharyngioma. *Eur J Endocrinol.* 2008;159(Suppl 1):95–99.

22. Teramoto A, Hirakawa K, Sanno N, Osamura Y. Incidental pituitary lesions in 1,000 unselected autopsy specimens. *Radiology.* 1994;193(1):161–64.

23. Larkin S, Ansorge O. Development and microscopic anatomy of the pituitary gland. In: Feingold KR, Anawalt B, Boyce A, Chrousos G, de Herder WW, Dhatariya K, et al., editors. *Endotext.* South Dartmouth, MA: MDText.com; 2017.

24. Kim E. Symptomatic Rathke cleft cyst: Clinical features and surgical outcomes. *World Neurosurg.* 2012;78(5):527–34.

25. Martinez Santos J, Hannay M, Olar A, Eskandari R. Rathke's cleft cyst apoplexy in two teenage sisters. *Pediatr Neurosurg.* 2019;54(6):428–35.

26. Amhaz HH, Chamoun RB, Waguespack SG, Shah K, McCutcheon IE. Spontaneous involution of Rathke cleft cysts: Is it rare or just underreported?: Report of 9 cases. *J Neurosurg.* 2010;112(6):1327–32.

Pituitary infiltrative and inflammatory disorders

OKSANA SYMCZYK

KEY POINTS

- Hypophysitis is an infiltrative or inflammatory disorder of the pituitary that can lead to anterior and posterior pituitary hormone deficits.
- Signs and symptoms of hypophysitis include headache, visual field disturbances, and cranial nerve palsies.

- Lymphocytic hypophysitis can develop during pregnancy and the early postpartum period.
- Treatment of hypophysitis during pregnancy involves thyroid hormone and glucocorticoid replacement. High doses of steroids are reserved for those experiencing severe headaches or visual deficits.

EPIDEMIOLOGY

- Lymphocytic hypophysitis is rare, occurring in approximately 1 per 9 million cases.[1]
- Lymphocytic hypophysitis is the most common primary infiltrative hypophysitis and affects females more than males in a 3:1 predominance.[2,3]
- More than half of women who develop lymphocytic hypophysitis present during pregnancy, typically in the last months of gestation or in the first several months postpartum.[3-8]
- Although both granulomatous and xanthomatous hypophysitis occur more frequently in women, neither form has been associated with onset during pregnancy.[9-11]
- IgG4-related (plasmacytic) hypophysitis occurs more frequently in men. It tends to develop at a more advanced age and does not have a known association with pregnancy.[12]

PATHOPHYSIOLOGY

- Infiltration and inflammation of the pituitary may develop primarily or secondarily from:
  - Lymphocytic infiltration
  - Granulomatous infiltration by giant cells and histiocytes
    - Associated with tuberculosis, sarcoidosis, granulomatosis with polyangiitis, medications such as ribavirin and α-interferon
  - Xanthomatous infiltration by foamy histiocytes
  - Plasma cell infiltration
  - Other:
    - Iron deposition due to hemochromatosis
    - Tumors including germinomas
    - CTLA-4 or PD-1 immunotherapy
    - Infections including mycotic infections or syphilis

DOI: 10.1201/9781003027577-30

- Sub-classification is dependent on the involved pituitary segment:
  - Anterior pituitary: Lymphocytic adenohypophysitis (LAH)
  - Posterior pituitary: Lymphocytic infundibular neurohypophysitis (LINH)
  - Mixed: Lymphocytic infundibular panhypophysitis (LPH)
- Hypophysitis results in destruction of the pituitary gland, with varying degrees of pituitary hormone deficiency.
- Enlargement of the pituitary gland due to infiltration and inflammation leads to[3]:
  - Headache
  - Visual field deficits
  - Cranial nerve III, IV, or VI palsies
  - Very rarely carotid artery occlusion
- Lymphocytic hypophysitis
  - Most common primary hypophysitis
  - An immune-mediated disorder characterized by infiltration of the pituitary gland by lymphocytes, mostly T-cells
  - Typically associated with other autoimmune disorders such as systemic lupus erythematosus, Sjögren syndrome, Hashimoto's thyroiditis, and Addison's disease [2,8,13]
  - No adverse effects on the fetus or gestational outcomes have been reported.[14]

DIAGNOSIS

- Typical presentation includes symptoms of hypopituitarism and/or symptoms of mass lesion such as headache and visual field deficits.
- Infiltrative pituitary disorders are more likely to cause diabetes insipidus in comparison to mass lesions. Diabetes insipidus should be suspected if symptoms include excessive thirst and urination significantly beyond that often experienced during pregnancy.
- Biochemical testing may reveal deficiencies in any or all of the following hormones:
  - Insulin-like growth factor 1 (IGF-1) as a measure of growth hormone
  - Thyroid-stimulating hormone (TSH) with concomitant free thyroxine (T4)
  - 8 AM plasma or serum cortisol
  - Prolactin

- Imaging
  - MRI without gadolinium is the imaging modality of choice to evaluate the sella in pregnancy.
  - Imaging appearance[2,15]:
    - Thickening of the pituitary stalk without deviation
    - Symmetrical pituitary enhancement
    - Loss of the neurohypophyseal "bright spot"
- Definitive diagnosis
  - Pituitary biopsy, although not routinely performed in pregnancy

TREATMENT

- Formal visual field examination is recommended for pregnant patients noting visual disturbances or if imaging suggests proximity to the optic chiasm.
- Conservative management during pregnancy is recommended.
- If present, adrenal insufficiency and hypothyroidism should be treated with glucocorticoids and levothyroxine, respectively.
- Initiate high dose steroids if there is progressive deterioration of vision, mass effect, or neurologic impairment.[16] Some centers use prednisone 60 mg/day or dexamethasone 8–10 mg/day; however, there is no consensus on dose or length of treatment as data is limited.[17]
- In refractory cases with severe symptoms, surgery for debulking may be considered but there is no reliable data regarding surgical management of hypophysitis during pregnancy.[3]

REFERENCES

1. Diego E, et al. A case report of lymphocytic hypophysitis related to pregnancy. *Open J Endocr Metab Dis.* 2015;5(12):1–6.
2. Bellastella A, Bizzarro A, Coronella C, Bellastella G, Sinisi AA, De Bellis A. Lymphocytic hypophysitis: A rare or underestimated disease? *Eur J Endocrinol.* 2003;149(5):363–76.
3. Faje A. Hypophysitis: Evaluation and management. *Clin Diabetes Endocrinol.* 2016;2(15):1–8.
4. Beressi N, Beressi JP, Cohen R, Modigliani E. Lymphocytic hypophysitis. A review

of 145 cases. *Ann Med Interne (Paris)*. 1999;150(4):327–41.

5. Kidd D, Wilson P, Unwin B, Dorward N. Lymphocytic hypophysitis presenting early in pregnancy. *J Neurol*. 2003;250(11): 1385–87.

6. Hashimoto K, Takao T, Makino S. Lymphocytic adenohypophysitis and lymphocytic infundibuloneurohypophysitis. *Endocr J*. 1997;44(1):1–10.

7. Caturegli P, Lupi I, Landek-Salgado M, Kimura H, Rose NR. Pituitary autoimmunity: 30 years later. *Autoimmun Rev*. 2008;7(8):631–37.

8. Caturegli P, Newschaffer C, Olivi A, Pomper MG, Burger PC, Rose NR. Autoimmune hypophysitis. *Endocr Rev*. 2005;26:599–614.

9. Hunn BHM, Martin WG, Simpson S Jr, Mclean CA. Idiopathic granulomatous hypophysitis: A systematic review of 82 cases in the literature. *Pituitary*. 2014;17(4):357–65.

10. Folkerth RD, Price DL Jr, Schwartz M, Black PM, De Girolami U. Xanthomatous hypophysitis. *Am J Surg Pathol*. 1998;22(6):736–41.

11. Hanna B, Li YM, Beutler T, Goyal P, Hall WA. Xanthomatous hypophysitis. *J Clin Neurosci*. 2015;22(7):1091–97.

12. Shimatsu A, Oki Y, Fujisawa I, Sano T. Pituitary and stalk lesions (infundibulo-hypophysitis) associated with immunoglobulin G4-related systemic disease: An emerging clinical entity. *Endocr J*. 2009;56(9):1033–41.

13. Landek-Salgado MA, Gutenberg A, Lupi I, Kimura H, Mariotti S, Rose NR, et al. Pregnancy, postpartum autoimmune thyroiditis, and autoimmune hypophysitis: Intimate relationships. *Autoimmun Rev*. 2010;9(3):153–57.

14. Biswas M, Thackare H, Jones MK, Bowen-Simpkins P. Lymphocytic hypophysitis and headache in pregnancy. *BJOG*. 2002;109(10):1184–86.

15. Sato N, Sze G, Endo K. Hypophysitis: Endocrinologic and dynamic MR findings. *AJNR Am J Neuroradiol*. 1998;19(3):439–44.

16. Reusch JE-B, Kleinschmidt-DeMasters BK, Lillehei KO, Rappe D, Gutierrez-Hartmann A. Preoperative diagnosis of lymphocytic hypophysitis (adenohypophysitis) unresponsive to short course dexamethasone: Case report. *Neurosurgery*. 1992;30(2):268–71.

17. Funazaki S, Yamada H, Hara K, Ishikawa S-E. Spontaneous pregnancy after full recovery from hypopituitarism caused by lymphocytic hypophysitis. *Endocrinol Diabetes Metab Case Rep* [Internet]. 2018. Available from: http://dx.doi.org/10.1530/edm-18-0081

5g

Diabetes insipidus

ADNAN HAIDER

- Central and nephrogenic diabetes insipidus (DI) can present prior to or during pregnancy.
- Gestational DI is specific to pregnancy and resolves following delivery.
- Plasma sodium and osmolality levels are reduced during pregnancy.
- The threshold of anti-diuretic hormone (ADH) release is reset to a lower concentration during pregnancy.
- Desmopressin (DDAVP) use is safe during pregnancy and lactation.

EPIDEMIOLOGY

- Diabetes insipidus (DI) is prevalent in approximately 2–4/100,000 pregnancies.[1-4] This includes central, nephrogenic, or gestational DI.
- The incidence of DI may be growing due to increased awareness of this condition.[1,5]
- Gestational DI is usually self-limited without major maternal or fetal morbidity or mortality risks; however, it can sometimes be the initial sign of developing liver dysfunction and can be associated with preeclampsia.

PATHOPHYSIOLOGY

- ADH is produced in the supraoptic and paraventricular nuclei and migrates down the pituitary stalk into the posterior pituitary where the hormone is stored.
- ADH is secreted from the posterior pituitary in response to increasing plasma osmolality, as sensed by osmoreceptors in the anterior pituitary, and to decreasing circulating volume,

as sensed by baroreceptors at the carotid artery bifurcation.[5]

- Physiologic changes during pregnancy:
  - The set-point of the osmoregulatory system is reduced during pregnancy. As a result, the threshold for ADH secretion is reduced and production of ADH rises; however, the net circulating levels are similar to the nonpregnant state due to breakdown of ADH by placental vasopressinase as discussed below.[6]
  - The threshold for thirst decreases, mediated by human chorionic gonadotropin (hCG).[7,8] This results in decreased plasma sodium concentrations by approximately 5 mEq/L and reduced plasma osmolality by approximately 10 mOsm/kg.[9]
  - The placenta secretes an enzyme called vasopressinase which inactivates ADH. This leads to a markedly shortened half-life of ADH, up to 4-fold faster clearance.[10]
  - In normal pregnancy, there is a consequent 4-fold increase in ADH production by hypothalamic nuclei. This rise in ADH

DOI: 10.1201/9781003027577-31

offsets the polyuria that commonly develops during pregnancy as a result of volume expansion, increased GFR, and clearance rate of ADH.

- The concentration of vasopressinase increases proportionally with the weight of the placental mass. Vasopressinase is initially measurable by week 10 of gestation and achieves maximal levels in the third trimester, with a 300-fold increase.[11]
- Vasopressinase levels decrease after delivery, with a reduction of 25% per day postpartum.[12]

- DI is the consequence of hormonal and chemical abnormalities that result in the production of a large volume of urine (polyuria) that is dilute (hypotonic).
- DI can develop prior to or during pregnancy. In some cases, preexisting DI is unmasked during pregnancy.
- ADH maintains normal serum osmolality by limiting the amount of free water excreted.
- Deficiency in the production of ADH by the hypothalamus or impairment of the release of ADH by the pituitary leads to central DI as free water is excreted into the urine in an uncontrolled manner.
- If hypothalamic and pituitary functions are intact with appropriate production and release of ADH, nephrogenic DI may still occur if the kidneys are unresponsive to the effects of the ADH.
- Gestational DI develops during pregnancy through the actions of placental vasopressinase which causes accelerated metabolism and transient deficiency of ADH. Vasopressinase is metabolized by the liver, therefore women with known hepatic dysfunction or who are at risk for hepatic dysfunction should be monitored for development of gestational DI. Conversely, women who are diagnosed with gestational DI should be evaluated for underlying hepatic dysfunction.[13] Other risk factors for the development of gestational DI include preeclampsia, HELLP syndrome, and twin pregnancies.[14]
- If a patient cannot drink enough water to compensate for renal water losses, the blood will become hypertonic and hypernatremia develops.
- For a summary of the characteristics of polydipsia and polyuria syndromes in pregnancy, see Table 5g.1.

DIAGNOSIS

- The initial step in diagnosing DI is to establish polyuria:
  - 24-hour urine collection while the patient is drinking ad lib
  - Interpretation: >50 mL/kg/day or >3 L/day of urine output without glucosuria
  - Polyuria can also result from uncontrolled hyperglycemia secondary to diabetes mellitus so a urine dipstick should be performed to rule out glucosuria
- Additional labs suggestive of DI in pregnancy:
  - Serum sodium ≥140 mEq/L
  - Serum osmolality ≥280 mOsm/kg
  - Urine osmolality <300 mOsm/kg
- Measurement of serum ADH has little utility because placental vasopressinase leads to undetectable ADH concentrations. Copeptin is a preprohormone of ADH which is secreted in similar concentrations to ADH, however is not as susceptible to the actions of vasopressinase. Therefore, measurement of copeptin may be useful to help distinguish central from gestational DI, although data is lacking.[6,15]
- Water deprivation testing
  - While dynamic testing using a water-restriction test is critical to the diagnosis of DI in the nonpregnant patient, this procedure should be limited in pregnancy due to increased risks of hypernatremia and uteroplacental insufficiency.[6,9]
  - If dynamic testing with water deprivation is necessary:
    - Perform in the hospital setting with close maternal and fetal monitoring
    - Must have confirmed polyuria on 24-hour urine collection
    - If serum sodium is >143 mEq/L, give 10 mcg intranasal or 4 mcg subcutaneous or intravenous DDAVP without water restriction.
    - If serum sodium is normal, proceed with water restriction.
      - Once the labs indicate mild hyperosmolality (serum sodium 143–146 mEq/L or plasma osmolality 290–295 mOsm/kg), measure the urine osmolality.
      - Then administer 10 mcg intranasal or 4 mcg subcutaneous or intravenous DDAVP.

Table 5g.1 Characteristics of polydipsia-polyuria syndromes during pregnancy and the immediate postpartum period

	Primary polydipsia	Gestational DI	Central DI	Nephrogenic DI
Pathophysiology	Habitual water intoxication	Increased placental vasopressinase-mediated clearance of ADH	Decreased secretory reserve of ADH	Renal resistance to ADH
Underlying causes or associations	Previously undiagnosed schizophrenia, anxiety disorders	May be associated with preeclampsia or liver abnormalities	Infiltrative processes, prior neurosurgery, idiopathic	Hypokalemia, hypercalcemia, lithium toxicity, hereditary gene mutation
Resolution following delivery	No	Yes	No	No
Recurrence with subsequent pregnancy	Possible	No	Yes[a]	Yes
Management	Psychiatry referral	Responsive to DDAVP	Responsive to DDAVP	Resistant to DDAVP, drink to thirst, consider thiazide diuretic or NSAIDs after delivery

[a] Lymphocytic hypophysitis is not expected to recur with subsequent pregnancies.

- Measure urine osmolality and urine volume every 30 minutes for a total of 2 hours
- Interpretation: An increase in urine osmolality to greater than 300 mOsm/kg is consistent with gestational or central DI

TREATMENT

- Central or gestational diabetes insipidus
  - Both central and gestational DI can be treated with DDAVP.
  - DDAVP
    - Vasopressin analog that is resistant to vasopressinase
    - Pregnancy category B
    - Selectively activates nonpressor V2 receptor, thus avoiding stimulation of blood pressure or uterine contractions[16,17]
    - Half-life of 12 hours
    - Can be administered intranasally, orally, intravenously, intramuscularly, or subcutaneously
      - Parenteral DDAVP is 10 times more potent than intranasal and 100 times more potent than oral formulations (Table 5g.2).
    - Starting dose: 10 mcg intranasal or 0.05 mg oral DDAVP at bedtime
    - Dosing can be titrated to relieve polyuria and maintain normal pregnancy serum sodium levels 133–140 mEq/L
- If the patient is hypernatremic, correct the sodium by replacing free water orally or intravenously.

Table 5g.2 DDAVP conversion chart

Subcutaneous or intramuscular	Intranasal	Oral
1 mcg	10 mcg	100 mcg (or 0.1 mg)

- Nephrogenic DI
  - DDAVP is ineffective, as there is resistance to ADH at the level of the kidneys.
  - Encourage drinking to thirst to avoid development of hypernatremia.
  - NSAIDs and thiazide diuretics have been used in nonpregnant patients but are not recommended in pregnancy.[18]

REFERENCES

1. Hime MC, Richardson JA. Diabetes insipidus and pregnancy. Case report, incidence and review of literature. *Obstet Gynecol Surv*. 1978; 33: 375–379.
2. Chanson P, Salenave S. Diabetes insipidus and pregnancy. *Ann Endocrinol (Paris)*. 2016; 77(2): 135–138.
3. Kondo T, Nakamura M, Kitano S, et al. The clinical course and pathophysiological investigation of adolescent gestational diabetes insipidus: A case report. *BMC Endocr Disord*. 2018; 18(1): 4.
4. Quigley J, Shelton C, Issa B, Sripada S. Diabetes insipidus in pregnancy. *Obstet Gynecol*. 2018; 20: 41–48.
5. Robertson GL. Physiology of ADH secretion. *Kidney Int suppl*. 1987; 21: S20–S26.
6. Bichard LK, Torpy DJ. Diabetes insipidus complicating apoplexy during pregnancy: The potential use of copeptin. *Intern Med J*. 2020; 50(7): 877–879.
7. Davison JM, Sheils EA, Philips PR. Serial evaluation of vasopressin release and thirst in human pregnancy. Role of HCG in the osmoregulatory changes of gestation. *J Clin Invest*. 1988; 81: 798–806.
8. Lindheimer MD, Barron WM, Davidson JM. Osmoregulation of thirst and vasopressin release in pregnancy. *Am J Physiology*. 1989; 257: F159–F169.
9. Lindheimer MD. Polyuria and pregnancy: Its cause, its danger. *Obstet Gynecol*. 2005; 105: 1171–1172.
10. Durr JA, Hoggard JG, Hunt JM, Schrier RW. Diabetes insipidus in pregnancy associated with abnormally high vasopressinase activity. *N Engl J Med*. 1987; 316; 1070–1074.
11. Davison JM, Sheills EA, Philips PR. Barron WM, Lindheimer MD. Metabolic clearance of vasopressinase in human pregnancy. *Am J physiol*. 1993; 264: F348–F353.
12. Page EW. The value of plasma pitocinase determinations in obstetrics. *Am J Obstet Gynecol*. 1946; 52: 1014–1022.
13. Marques P, Gunawardana K, Grossman A. Transient diabetes insipidus in pregnancy. *Endocrinol Diabetes Metab Case Rep*. 2015; 2015: 150078.
14. Gambito R, Chan M, Sheta M, et al. Gestational diabetes insipidus associated with HELLP syndrome: A case report. *Case Rep Nephrol*. 2012; 2012: 640365.
15. Refardt J, Christ-Crain M. Copeptin-based diagnosis of diabetes insipidus. *Swiss Med Wkly*. 2020; 150: w20237.
16. Ananthakrishnan S. Diabetes insipidus in pregnancy: Etiology, evaluation and management. *Endo Prac*. 2009; 15(4): 377–381.
17. Ray JG. DDAVP use during pregnancy: An analysis of its safety for mother and child. *Obstet Gynecol*. 1998; 53: 450–455.
18. Hague WM. Diabetes insipidus in pregnancy. *Obstet Med*. 2009 Dec; 2(4): 138–141.

Hyponatremia in pregnancy

ANTHONY PARRAVANI AND BETHANY PELLEGRINO

KEY POINTS

- Mild, euvolemic hyponatremia is common in pregnancy secondary to a reset osmostat, which is a change in the set point of anti-diuretic hormone (ADH) release and stimulation of thirst.
- The syndrome of inappropriate ADH (SIADH) can occur in pregnancy, typically associated with nonosmotic stimuli such as hypovolemia, nausea, and pain, promoting the release of ADH.
- Excess water intake may be the most common reason for hyponatremia during labor.

- Judicious use of oral and intravenous hypotonic fluids, careful monitoring of sodium levels with oxytocin administration, and correction of potential nonosmotic stimuli for ADH release are needed to prevent severe, symptomatic hyponatremia.
- Avoidance of overly rapid correction of hyponatremia is necessary to avoid serious complications such as osmotic demyelination syndrome, formerly known as central pontine myelinolysis.

EPIDEMIOLOGY

- While no incidence data is available for mild hyponatremia in pregnancy, the condition is felt to be very common and benign.[1]
- More severe hyponatremia such as what has been described in association with SIADH is far less common.[2] Various case reports of SIADH being associated with preeclampsia still describe a relatively rare occurrence.[3]

PATHOPHYSIOLOGY

Nonpregnant state, maintenance of serum osmolality and sodium:

- Under nonpregnant conditions, serum osmolality is maintained within a narrow range of 275–295 mOsm/L.

- Any changes in serum osmolality are sensed by osmoreceptors which respond to correct the change.
  - An increase in serum osmolality by 1–2% results in the release of ADH from the posterior pituitary, which acts on the Arginine Vasopressin Receptor 2 (AVPR2) on the basolateral membrane of the collecting ducts in the kidneys. This leads to the upregulation of aquaporin 2 channels and increased water absorption by the kidneys.
  - Any increase in serum osmolality also stimulates the thirst center in the hypothalamus, resulting in water intake to assist in correction of the hypertonic state.[4]

Pregnant state:

- Mild hyponatremia is common in pregnancy.

DOI: 10.1201/9781003027577-32

- Beginning in early pregnancy and stabilizing by week 12 gestation, a reduction in plasma osmolality by approximately 10 mOsm/L and reduction in sodium by approximately 5 mmol/L occurs. These changes correct after delivery.[5,6]
- The kidney response to ADH compares to the nonpregnant state, but the maximum capacity to excrete a water load is about one-third of prepregnancy capacity.[7]
  - This state, characterized by an elevation of ADH at lower plasma osmolality, is sometimes referred to as a reset osmostat.
  - These changes are thought to be mediated by the fetal-placental unit.
- Vascular changes
  - Relative arterial underfilling during pregnancy contributes to mild hyponatremia.
  - Increased levels of estrogen and relaxin in pregnancy result in systemic vasodilation.
  - An incomplete increase in cardiac output and activation of the renin-angiotensin and sympathetic systems work to counteract this, yet the net effect is an overall drop in arterial blood pressure.
  - This leads to a nonosmotic stimulus for ADH release as well as the stimulation of thirst.[1]
- Vasopressinase
  - With numerous factors increasing the release of ADH during pregnancy, a significant alteration in the metabolism of ADH occurs.
  - The metabolism of ADH is mediated by the production of vasopressinase, an aminopeptide produced by placental trophoblasts that functions to degrade ADH.
  - Overproduction of vasopressinase has been described in a form of diabetes insipidus associated with pregnancy, wherein the depletion of ADH leads to excess free water loss, polyuria, and hypernatremia (see Chapter 5g).[8,9]
- SIADH
  - ADH release without appropriate osmotic triggers characterizes the syndrome of inappropriate secretion of ADH (SIADH).
  - The release of ADH in this scenario results in excess water retention.

- Excess water retention in turn is associated with a pressure natriuresis leading to both free water retention and sodium loss.
- Nonosmotic triggers in pregnancy-associated SIADH are pain, nausea, and fear.
- Serum sodium levels can significantly drop when the patient receives hypotonic fluids, with the inability to excrete free water.
- Several case reports of SIADH occurring with preeclampsia are in the literature, but it is not completely clear why this happens. Potentially, the combined effects of SIADH and low effective circulating volume with preeclampsia result in the severe hyponatremia described.[1,9,10]
- Other causes of severe hyponatremia in pregnancy:
  - Polydipsia can play a role in hyponatremia that develops in the pregnant patient, particularly in the peripartum phase.
    - Increased free water intake either due to stress or social encouragement may overcome the kidney's ability to excrete the water load.
  - The combined factors of increased ADH release due to pain or nausea and increased free water consumption have been described in pregnant patients with severe hyponatremia.
  - Hyponatremia during labor is now thought to be primarily associated with overdrinking.[2]
  - Oxytocin administration
    - Oxytocin is a hormone stored and released by the posterior pituitary, with a molecular structure similar to that of ADH.
    - Oxytocin can have an effect similar to ADH on water reabsorption in the kidneys.
    - Oxytocin is administered peripartum to stimulate uterine contractions during labor. Coupled with the administration of hypotonic fluids, oxytocin infusions can cause significant hyponatremia.
      - Current recommendations suggest the infusion of oxytocin in Ringers Lactate or 0.9% normal saline with close monitoring of sodium levels to prevent severe hyponatremia.[2]

DIAGNOSIS

Signs and symptoms:

- Dependent on severity and duration of the hyponatremia
  - Sodium 130–135 mEq/L: No symptoms are generally reported.
  - Sodium <130 mEq/L: Headache, nausea, dizziness, drowsiness, seizure, and coma.
  - Symptoms are often vague, nonspecific, and can be associated with preeclampsia or parturition, thus effective identification is reliant on a high index of suspicion.[2,3]
- Severe hyponatremia is associated with:
  - Pregnancy risks: Preeclampsia
  - Fetal risks: Oligohydramnios, polyhydramnios, intrauterine growth restriction, and seizures[3]
- With mild hyponatremia in pregnancy (serum sodium ≥130 mEq/L), further workup is not considered necessary unless the patient is symptomatic.
- With more severe hyponatremia, workup is similar to that in the nonpregnant patient
  - Assess volume status to delineate hypovolemic, euvolemic, and hypervolemic causes[1,3]
  - Measure serum osmolality to rule out pseudohyponatremia or hyperosmolar hyponatremia
  - Measure urine osmolality and random urine sodium to evaluate hypoosmolar hyponatremia:
    - Assess patient's medications
    - Assess patient's kidney function and GFR
    - Assess for undiagnosed or untreated adrenal insufficiency or hypothyroidism
- Laboratory findings
  - Reset osmostat
    - Low serum osmolality
    - Low urine osmolality
    - Variable urine sodium
  - SIADH
    - Low serum osmolality in a euvolemic patient
    - Urine osmolality >100 mOsm/L due to ADH secretion despite hypoosmolality
    - Urine sodium >40 mmol/L, indicating pressure natriuresis

- Note: Plasma ADH levels are not typically followed as it is difficult to measure clinically and the urine osmolality can be used as a surrogate marker of ADH release.[3,7]

TREATMENT

- Mild hyponatremia of pregnancy due to reset osmostat
  - No treatment is required
  - Fluid restriction and salt supplementation are unlikely to correct sodium levels due to the underlying factor being a change in the set point for ADH release
- SIADH
  - Requires close monitoring to avoid over-correction
  - Fluid restriction and salt supplementation are the initial treatments in those without symptoms[5]
  - More aggressive management with 3% saline is warranted with severe hyponatremia with symptoms[3]
  - Vasopressin antagonists (Vaptans) used for management of hyponatremia have not been studied in pregnancy, but risk of fetal harm is thought to be low based on animal data[9]
- Polydipsia
  - Free water restriction should be an adequate treatment[2]
- Oxytocin
  - During oxytocin administration, monitor serum sodium levels
  - Avoid use of hypotonic fluids with the oxytocin infusion[2]
- Treatment of hyponatremia should be such that rapid correction is avoided
  - A rise in serum sodium no more than 8–10 mmol/L over 24 hours is the goal
  - Rapid overcorrection can result in the devastating osmotic demyelination syndrome (central pontine myelinolysis)[3,4]

REFERENCES

1. Pazhayattil GS, Rastegar A, Brewster UC. Approach to the Diagnosis and Treatment of Hyponatremia in Pregnancy. *Am J Kidney Dis.* 2015; 65(4):623–627.
2. Jellema J, Balt J, Broeze K, Scheele F, Weijmer M. Hyponatremia during

Pregnancy. *Internet J Gynecol Obstet*. 2008; 12(1):1–6.

3. Traill C, Halpern SH. Syndrome of Inappropriate Antidiuretic Hormone. In: Mankowitz S. (ed.) *Consults on Obstetric Anesthesiology*. Springer, Cham. 2018: 569–570.

4. Rose BD. New Approach to Disturbances in the Plasma Sodium Concentration. *Am J Med*. 1986; 81(6):1033–1040.

5. Feder J, Gomez JM, Serra-Aguirre F, Musso CG. Reset Osmostat. *Indian J Nephrol*. 2019; 29(4):232–234.

6. Sutton AL, Schonnholzer K, Kassen BO. Transient Syndrome of Inappropriate Hormone Secretion During Pregnancy. *Am J Kidney Dis*. 1993; 21(4):444–445.

7. Moen V, Brudin L, Rundgren M, Irestedt L. Hyponatremia Complicating Labour—rare or unrecognized? A prospective observational study. *BJOG*. 2009; 116:552–561.

8. Kondo T, Nakamura M, Kitano S, et al. The Clinical Course and Pathophysiological Investigation of Adolescent Gestational Diabetes Insipidus: A Case Report. *BMC Endocr Disord*. 2018; 18(4):1–8.

9. Marques P, Gunnawardana K, Grossman A. Transient Diabetes Insipidus. *Endocrinol Diabetes Metab Case Rep*. 2015; 2015:150078.

10. Sardidogan E, Kirbas A, Elmas B, Caglar T. The Role of Hyponatremia in Preeclampsia. *Medicine Science*. 2017; 6(3):592–597.

Pituitary emergencies: Sheehan's syndrome and apoplexy

JESSICA PERINI, NADIA BARGHOUTHI, AND GAYATRI JAISWAL

KEY POINTS

- Pituitary apoplexy consists of a potentially life-threatening hemorrhage into the pituitary gland.
- Sheehan's syndrome develops from acute infarction of the pituitary gland following postpartum hemorrhage.
- Adrenal crisis is the most immediate life-threatening consequence of pituitary damage.
- Central hypothyroidism also develops but the symptoms and signs can take weeks to manifest.

- After pituitary infarction or hemorrhage, one or more pituitary hormones may be deficient and the degree of deficiency can vary from person to person.
- Inability to nurse is often the first sign of pituitary insufficiency in the postpartum period.
- Both Sheehan's syndrome and pituitary apoplexy require prompt diagnosis, immediate treatment with glucocorticoids, neurosurgical consultation, and long-term monitoring of pituitary hormone function.

EPIDEMIOLOGY

- The prevalence and incidence of Sheehan's syndrome vary significantly from country to country, but the syndrome is rare overall. In developed countries, rates vary from 0.2 to 5 of 100,000 women.[1]
- Sheehan's syndrome is an uncommon cause of hypopituitarism. Approximately 0.5% of hypopituitarism cases in women are attributable to Sheehan's syndrome.[2]
- Up to 56% of women who develop hypopituitarism due to Sheehan's syndrome lose function of all anterior pituitary hormones, while 44% experience partial hypopituitarism.[3]

- Anterior pituitary hormones are most commonly affected in Sheehan's syndrome but posterior pituitary hormones are occasionally involved, with cases of isolated anti-diuretic hormone (ADH), also known as vasopressin, deficiency and resultant diabetes insipidus reported in the literature.[4,5]
- An inability to lactate is often the first symptom noted in those with Sheehan's syndrome.[6]
- Pituitary apoplexy in pregnancy has a prevalence of approximately 1 in 10,000.[7]
- Of women diagnosed with pituitary apoplexy during pregnancy, 42–47% had known pituitary lesions prior to pregnancy.[7]

DOI: 10.1201/9781003027577-33

PATHOPHYSIOLOGY

Sheehan's syndrome

- Acute blood loss during labor, delivery, and the postpartum period can lead to severe hypotension and resultant ischemic injury to the pituitary gland.
- Several factors allow the pituitary gland to be more susceptible to injury during this time[8]:
  - Pituitary gland enlarges during pregnancy due in part to hyperplasia of lactotrophs
  - Larger size of the pituitary gland increases metabolic needs of the gland, yet vascular supply cannot increase significantly due to the physical confines of the gland in the sella turcica and low pressure of the feeding vessels.
- Risk factors that may increase risk of developing Sheehan's syndrome[8]:
  - Disseminated intravascular coagulation
  - Anemia
  - Uterine atony
  - Vasospasm
  - Thrombosis history
  - Advanced maternal age
- Ischemic injury with subsequent necrosis may affect one, several, or all of the pituitary hormones including anterior and posterior pituitary hormones.
  - Anterior pituitary hormones include:
    - Adrenocorticotropic hormone (ACTH)
    - Thyroid-stimulating hormone (TSH)
    - Prolactin
    - Luteinizing hormone (LH)
    - Follicle-stimulating hormone (FSH)
    - Growth hormone (GH)
  - Posterior pituitary hormones include:
    - Oxytocin
    - ADH
- Necrosis of the corticotrophs of the pituitary will impair secretion of ACTH, which stimulates the production of cortisol by the adrenal glands.
  - If the ACTH deficiency is severe and acute, adrenal insufficiency will rapidly develop and, if not identified and treated quickly, may progress to a potentially fatal adrenal crisis with severe hypotension, hypoglycemia, hyponatremia, and shock.
  - If the corticotrophs are only mildly damaged, the deficiency of ACTH may not be immediately obvious and longer-term symptoms of adrenal insufficiency such as lethargy, loss of appetite, weight loss, and diarrhea may occur gradually.
- Necrosis of the thyrotrophs of the pituitary will impair secretion of TSH, which stimulates the production of thyroid hormone by the thyroid gland.
  - Symptoms of hypothyroidism will not be apparent in the immediate postpartum period due to the long half-life of thyroid hormone (7 days).
  - Symptoms of hypothyroidism include fatigue, weight gain, trouble concentrating, cold intolerance, and constipation. Severe symptoms include bradycardia, hypothermia, and altered mental status.
- Necrosis of the lactotrophs of the pituitary will impair production of prolactin.
  - The primary symptom of low prolactin is an inability to lactate. This is often the first indication of pituitary hypofunction in women with Sheehan's syndrome.
- Necrosis of the gonadotrophs leads to impaired production of FSH and LH, which are essential in ovarian function and fertility.
  - Lack of menstruation and infertility are common consequences of Sheehan's syndrome.
  - After years of low estrogen due to central hypogonadism, women develop an increased risk of osteoporosis.
- Necrosis of the somatotrophs of the pituitary impairs production of growth hormone.
  - Growth hormone deficiency can lead to fatigue, decrease in muscle or lean body mass, and a diminished sense of well-being.
- Necrosis of the posterior pituitary may affect ADH function and lead to central diabetes insipidus with excessive urination and thirst. Oxytocin deficiency will impair the ability to breastfeed.
- Symptoms of hypopituitarism may develop immediately or slowly over months to decades.

Pituitary apoplexy

- During pregnancy, the prolactin-producing lactotroph cells of the pituitary expand in both size and number.

- By approximately three days after delivery, the pituitary gland may be up to 136% of its prepregnancy size.[7]
- The enlarged gland and the pregnant state lead to an increased risk for ischemia, thrombosis, and bleeding.
- Pregnant women who develop pituitary apoplexy may have a previously diagnosed or an undiagnosed pituitary tumor.
- As lactotrophs expand into or adjacent to a pre-existing pituitary tumor, there is an increased risk of hemorrhage.
- Sudden hemorrhage into the pituitary gland causes swelling and destruction to the gland which may lead to deficiency of any or all of the pituitary hormones.

DIAGNOSIS

- Pituitary apoplexy can present with severe, sudden headache, vision changes, lethargy, nausea, and vomiting. Both Sheehan's syndrome and pituitary apoplexy can present with symptoms of adrenal insufficiency and inability to lactate.
- Adrenal insufficiency
  - If postpartum hypotension persists despite adequate fluid resuscitation, suspicion for acute adrenal insufficiency should be high.
  - Other symptoms to suggest adrenal insufficiency include hyponatremia, fever, nausea, vomiting, diarrhea, extreme fatigue, mental status changes, polyuria, or new-onset congestive heart failure.
  - A cortisol level <5 mcg/dL (<3 mcg/dL in some guidelines) indicates adrenal insufficiency.
  - When measuring a cortisol level, the test must be performed on a blood sample drawn prior to administration of glucocorticoids.
  - A low cortisol level will aid in the diagnosis of adrenal insufficiency, but treatment with glucocorticoids should not be delayed while awaiting results of the blood test.
- Evaluation for central hypothyroidism involves measuring a TSH with a concomitant free T4.
  - A low free T4 with a low or inappropriately normal TSH confirms the diagnosis.
  - Due to the long half-life of thyroid hormone, labs will not necessarily demonstrate hypothyroidism for at least 4–6 weeks.
- Lactation failure in the immediate postpartum period or after months should raise suspicion for Sheehan's syndrome.
  - Hypoprolactinemia can be diagnosed with a low prolactin level.
- Imaging:
  - MRI of the sella can be performed with gadolinium if postpartum and without gadolinium in pregnant patients.
  - MRI of the brain with pituitary protocol demonstrates empty sella in approximately 70% of those with Sheehan's syndrome. For pituitary apoplexy, hemorrhage into the sella can be seen.

TREATMENT

- Prompt treatment of hormone deficiencies can reduce mortality and morbidity.
- Patients with Sheehan's syndrome who develop pituitary hormone deficiencies are not expected to recover pituitary function over time.
- As adrenal insufficiency can be life-threatening, cortisol should be replaced immediately.
  - See Chapters 4f and 4h for management of adrenal insufficiency and adrenal crisis, respectively.
  - Glucocorticoid administration should not be delayed while cortisol results are pending.
  - If a cortisol level drawn prior to the administration of any steroid medication indicates adequate adrenal function, the glucocorticoid can be discontinued.
- In patients with both central hypothyroidism and hypocortisolism, glucocorticoids should be replaced before initiation of thyroid hormone to reduce the risk of inducing an adrenal crisis.
  - Treatment of central hypothyroidism involves replacing thyroid hormone with levothyroxine at a starting dose of 1.6–1.7 mcg/kg/day.
  - Free T4 must be used to guide dosing of levothyroxine in central hypothyroidism, as TSH is unreliable in the setting of pituitary dysfunction.
- Hypogonadism should be treated with estrogen (plus progesterone in the presence of an intact

uterus) replacement therapy at physiologic doses until the patient reaches the standard age of menopause to minimize risk to bone health.

- Patients who wish to pursue subsequent pregnancies should be referred to reproductive specialists.
- Diabetes insipidus should be treated with desmopressin (DDAVP) (see Chapter 5g).
- Replacement of GH may be considered in patients with GH deficiency, although its use is still somewhat controversial (see Chapter 5c).
- Pituitary apoplexy
  - In addition to the hormone treatments discussed previously, neurosurgical consultation is recommended.
  - Dopamine agonist therapy with bromocriptine or cabergoline is sometimes useful to help with symptoms by shrinking lactotrophs and the size of the pituitary over time, however, will likely impair lactation.

REFERENCES

1. Ramiandrasoa C, et al. Delayed diagnosis of Sheehan's syndrome in a developed country: A retrospective cohort study. *Euro J Endocrinol.* 2013 Oct;169(4):431–438.

2. Genetu A, et al. A 45-year-old female patient with Sheehan's syndrome presenting with imminent adrenal crisis: A case report. *J Med Case Rep.* 2021;15:229.

3. Keleştimur F, et al. Sheehan's syndrome: Baseline characteristics and effect of 2 years of growth hormone replacement therapy in 91 patients in KIMS—Pfizer International Metabolic Database. *Eur J Endocrinol.* 2005 Apr;152(4):581–587.

4. Kumar S, et al. Sheehan syndrome presenting as central diabetes insipidus: A rare presentation of an uncommon disorder. *Endocr Pract.* 2011 Jan–Feb;17(1):108–114.

5. Laway BA, et al. Sheehan's syndrome with central diabetes insipidus. *Arq Bras Endocrinol Metabol.* 2011 Mar;55(2):171–174.

6. Schrager S, Sabo L. Sheehan syndrome: A rare complication of postpartum hemorrhage. *J Amer Brd Fam Prac.* 2001;14(5):389–391.

7. Grand'Maison S, et al. Pituitary apoplexy in pregnancy: A case series and literature review. *Obstet Med.* 2015 Dec;8(4):177–183.

8. Karaca Z, et al. Sheehan syndrome. *Nature Rev Dis Primers.* 2016 Dec;2:16092.

CHAPTER 6

Calcium and Metabolic Bone Disorders

Hypercalcemia and hyperparathyroidism

SHIRA B. EYTAN

KEY POINTS

- Diagnosis of primary hyperparathyroidism in pregnancy can be difficult due to overlap with common pregnancy symptoms.
- Physiologic changes in pregnancy such as decreased albumin levels and increased glomerular filtration rate can make calcium levels appear falsely lower. To accurately evaluate calcium levels in pregnancy, calcium should be adjusted for albumin or ionized calcium can be checked.
- Medical management of primary hyperparathyroidism is often acceptable during pregnancy, but both mother and neonate should have a close follow-up to avoid complications. If surgical treatment is necessary, second trimester is preferred.

EPIDEMIOLOGY

- Primary hyperparathyroidism (PHPT) is rarely diagnosed in pregnancy, with an incidence estimated to be around 1%. However, complications from this diagnosis are high, with approximately 67% maternal and 80% fetal or neonatal complication rates.[1]
- The prevalence may be higher; however, expansion of intravascular volume and decreases in serum albumin levels can mask hypercalcemia in pregnancy.[1,2] Therefore, diagnosis may be delayed in pregnancy as normal physiologic changes lower total calcium and parathyroid hormone (PTH) levels.
- In a series of 109 mothers with PHPT during pregnancy who were treated medically (N = 70) or surgically (N = 39), there was 53% incidence of neonatal complications and 16% incidence of neonatal deaths among medically-treated mothers, as opposed to 12.5% neonatal complications and 2.5% neonatal deaths in mothers who underwent parathyroidectomy.[3]

PATHOPHYSIOLOGY

Calcium homeostasis in pregnancy

- A term infant requires approximately 25–30 g of calcium, 20 g of phosphorus, and 0.8 g of magnesium for bone mineralization during fetal development.[2-4] At least 80% of these minerals are accumulated during the third trimester.[2] During pregnancy, intestinal calcium absorption doubles to meet fetal requirements, and during lactation, skeletal resorption increases to provide sufficient calcium for breast milk.
- Ionized calcium does not change throughout pregnancy even though the serum calcium drops approximately 10%.[2] Maternal calcium is transported through the placenta leading to higher fetal blood calcium concentrations of 0.5–1 mEq/L in comparison with maternal blood. This results in suppression of fetal PTH secretion until after delivery. When PHPT is present, there is further fetal PTH suppression

DOI: 10.1201/9781003027577-35

which increases risks of neonatal hypocalcemia and tetany after delivery.

- Parathyroid hormone-related peptide (PTHrP) is a prohormone that was first noted in tumors which led to hypercalcemia of malignancy. Its NH2-terminal has partial homology to PTH which enables it to activate the common PTH/PTHrP receptor and have identical functions as PTH. Normally, PTHrP is undetectable in adults, but in pregnancy, it increases, especially in the third trimester.[5]
  - Sources of PTHrP may include the placenta, parathyroid, breasts, amnion, and fetal tissue.
  - The rise in PTHrP likely contributes to the maintenance of ionized calcium, increased levels of calcitriol, and suppression of PTH during pregnancy.[2] It inhibits osteoclast-mediated bone resorption and may protect the maternal skeleton against excessive bone resorption during pregnancy.[5]
  - During lactation, PTHrP rises significantly and seems to be derived from breast tissue. It is released into milk at 10,000 times the levels seen in non-lactating controls or hypercalcemia of malignancy. The role of PTHrP during lactation is to stimulate resorption of calcium from the maternal skeleton, renal tubular reabsorption of calcium, and suppression of PTH.[5]
- PTH is suppressed to the lower end of normal (approximately 0–30% of nonpregnant values) in all three trimesters.[2] It reaches a trough in the low to normal range in the first trimester, sometimes dropping to undetectable range, then steadily increasing to normal throughout the pregnancy.[5] In some studies, PTH did not decline in pregnancy and was shown to rise in some cases, likely due to diets traditionally low in vitamin D or calcium and high in phytate (which blocks calcium absorption), provoking a compensatory secondary hyperparathyroidism in pregnancy.[2]
- During exclusive lactation, PTH remains low or undetectable then rises during weaning.[5]

Pathologic conditions

PRIMARY HYPERPARATHYROIDISM

- Although PHPT is common in the general population, it is rare in pregnancy, occurring in about 0.03% of women of reproductive age.[6] The diagnosis may be confounded by normal pregnancy-related decreases in serum albumin and PTH levels.
- The etiology of PHPT in pregnancy is similar to nonpregnant cases with single parathyroid adenomas as the most common cause followed by four gland hyperplasia.
- Symptoms overlap with common pregnancy symptoms such as nausea, vomiting, abdominal pain, renal colic, muscular weakness, skeletal pain, or fatigue. This overlap may delay diagnosis.
- Absorptive hypercalciuria of pregnancy predisposes to nephrolithiasis and is likely aggravated by PHPT. Pancreatitis may be the presenting manifestation in up to 15% of cases of PHPT in pregnancy and usually occurs during the second or third trimester.[5]
- Severe hypercalcemia or parathyroid crisis can occur during the third trimester or, more commonly, postpartum. Rapid transfer of calcium across the placenta during the third trimester may protect against maternal hypercalcemia, but this effect is abruptly lost after delivery of the placenta, thereby precipitating postpartum hypercalcemic crisis.[5]
- PHPT in pregnancy is associated with adverse outcomes such as stillbirth and neonatal death in 2% of cases and tetany in 15%. This is due to suppression of fetal and neonatal parathyroid glands which may be prolonged several months after delivery or, in some cases, lifelong.[7]
- Most cases of PHPT are sporadic, presenting with a single parathyroid adenoma. However, hereditary syndromes such as multiple endocrine neoplasia, familial hypocalciuric hypercalcemia (FHH), and jaw-tumor syndrome should be kept in mind. Though hereditary forms of PHPT usually correspond with multiglandular diseases, they may initially present with PHPT alone.

FAMILIAL HYPOCALCIURIC HYPERCALCEMIA

- FHH is an autosomal dominant condition caused by inactivating mutations in the calcium-sensing receptor (CASR), which lead to hypercalcemia, hypocalciuria, and high-normal or elevated PTH levels. It is asymptomatic and the elevation in calcium and PTH persists during pregnancy. However, during pregnancy, the increased intestinal calcium absorption may cause hypercalciuria which can complicate the diagnosis. Pregnancies in women with FHH are uneventful, but neonates may develop hypoparathyroidism in utero with increased calcium flux across the placenta, causing fetal parathyroid suppression which can last for several months after birth.[2] Thus, the newborn should be monitored for hypocalcemia.

PSEUDOHYPERPARATHYROIDISM

- Pseudohyperparathyroidism is defined as PTHrP-mediated hypercalcemia. Its occurrence during pregnancy confirms the potential physiologic importance of the breasts and placenta in contributing to the regulation of maternal mineral homeostasis. When the placenta is the cause, hypercalcemia usually corrects within hours of delivery, whereas production by the breasts is more likely to lead to sustained hypercalcemia after delivery.

DIAGNOSIS

- Symptoms that should raise suspicion for maternal PHPT include severe nausea or vomiting, peptic ulcer disease, pancreatitis, nephrolithiasis, or a history of spontaneous abortions or neonatal death. Symptoms of hypercalcemia are nonspecific and similar to many pregnancy-related symptoms.
  - Occasionally, some patients can present with confusion.
  - Nephrolithiasis is the most common finding in symptomatic patients with PHPT during pregnancy.[8]
  - A possible early symptom of gestational PHPT is hyperemesis gravidarum.[9]
  - Hypertension is present in 10% of cases.[10]
  - Fractures are uncommon but have been reported with more severe hyperparathyroidism and parathyroid carcinoma.[2]
- Diagnosis of PHPT can be made with elevated PTH and albumin-corrected or ionized calcium levels.
- During pregnancy, PTH should be measured only by two-site "intact" or "bio-intact" PTH assays for accuracy.
- Localization of a parathyroid adenoma may be difficult during pregnancy as radioisotope-labeled scans should be avoided. Neck

ultrasound can provide focal localization in a majority of cases but may lack sensitivity. Ten percent of cases involve 4-gland parathyroid hyperplasia so these cases along with ectopic parathyroid glands can make localization more difficult.

TREATMENT

- To prevent adverse outcomes, surgical treatment of PHPT is recommended during the second trimester to avoid complications of anesthesia and surgery during the first and third trimesters.[3]
- Conservative management, in addition to close follow-up until and after delivery, can be appropriate if the patient is asymptomatic. These measures are limited to hydration and electrolyte balance.
- Pharmacologic treatments of hypercalcemia have not been adequately studied nor approved in pregnancy. Clinical experience with pharmacologic therapies is limited to individual case reports so the relative benefits and risks of each option are not clear. Therefore, parathyroidectomy is the only definitive treatment of PHPT.
  - Calcitonin (pregnancy category B) does not cross the placenta and has been used in pregnancy to suppress bone resorption and promote urine calcium excretion. It may be used acutely and effectively in the short term but loses its efficacy due to tachyphylaxis.
  - Oral phosphate (pregnancy category C) has been used in pregnancy with modest efficacy to bind calcium. The most common side effects are diarrhea and hypokalemia.
  - Bisphosphonate therapy is contraindicated in pregnancy as these medications cross the placenta and may interfere with fetal endochondral bone development.[5]
  - Cinacalcet (pregnancy category C) has been used in pregnancy in at least 1 case.[5] This medication acts on the calcium receptor to suppress PTH and stimulate calcitonin, thereby lowering serum calcium levels. Its use in pregnancy is limited by the side effect of nausea. In addition, the calcium receptor is also expressed in the placenta and fetal parathyroid glands, so cinacalcet

may also suppress the fetal parathyroid glands, stimulate fetal calcitonin, and alter the rate of placental calcium transfer.

- High-dose magnesium also acts on the calcium receptor to decrease PTH and calcium.

- During surgery, intraoperative PTH monitoring increases cure rate success. In preparation for surgery, calcitonin may be used preoperatively along with intravenous fluid hydration, especially in cases of patients with severe hypercalcemia.[11] Postoperative monitoring of electrolytes is important. Calcium and vitamin D repletion after surgery to correct deficiencies is recommended, especially after removal of a large parathyroid adenoma to avoid hypocalcemia. Potassium and magnesium should also be monitored, as deficiency may exist but may not be detectable until the serum calcium has normalized.

- If medical management is pursued, there should be surveillance of maternal serum calcium and PTH during the pregnancy in addition to regular biophysical profiles of the fetus by ultrasonography.

- In the postpartum period, serum calcium levels increase after the placenta is delivered. Postpartum parathyroidectomy should be considered in cases that were medically managed during pregnancy.

- Following delivery, neonates should be monitored for hypocalcemia. The blood calcium normally decreases about 20% over the first 12 hours with the onset of breathing and rises to the normal range over the succeeding 24–48 hours.[5] Neonatal hypoparathyroidism caused by maternal hyperparathyroidism is usually transient and should be treated with calcium and calcitriol. Neonates should also be fed milk formulas high in calcium and low in phosphate to minimize the risk of hypocalcemia. Neonatal hypoparathyroidism may be permanent and thus ongoing surveillance should be performed.

- Lactation contributes significantly to bone resorption due to the combined effects of PTHrP and low estradiol; therefore, hypercalcemia can be expected to worsen in breastfeeding mothers.

- Potential maternal hypercalcemia should be considered when deciding between active monitoring versus postpartum parathyroidectomy.

REFERENCES

1. McCarthy A, Howarth S, Khoo S, et al. Management of Primary Hyperparathyroidism in Pregnancy: A Case Series. *Endocrinol Diabetes Metab Case Rep.* 2019;2019: 19–0039.

2. Kovacs CS. Maternal Mineral and Bone Metabolism During Pregnancy, Lactation, and Post-Weaning Recovery. *Physiol Rev.* 2016;96(2):449–547.

3. Beattie GC, Ravi NR, Lewis M, et al. Rare Presentation of Maternal Primary Hyperparathyroidism. *BMJ.* 2000;321(7255):223–224.

4. Kelly TR. Primary Hyperparathyroidism During Pregnancy. *Surgery.* 1991;110(6):1028–1034.

5. Truong MT, Lalakea ML, Robbins P, Friduss M. Primary Hyperparathyroidism in Pregnancy: A Case Series and Review. *Laryngoscope.* 2008;118(11):1966–1969.

6. Kovacs CS. Calcium and Bone Metabolism Disorders During Pregnancy and Lactation. *Endocrinol Metab Clin North Am.* 2011;40(4):795–826.

7. Hirsch D, Kopel V, Nadler V, Levy S, Toledano Y, Tsvetov G. Pregnancy Outcomes in Women with Primary Hyperparathyroidism. *J Clin Endocrinol Metab.* 2015;100(5):2115–2122.

8. Shangold MM, Dor N, Welt SI, Fleischman AR, Crenshaw MC Jr. Hyperparathyroidism and Pregnancy: A Review. *Obstet Gynecol Surv.* 1982;37(4):217–228.

9. Mestman JH. Parathyroid Disorders of Pregnancy. *Semin Perinatol.* 1998;22(6): 485–496.

10. Pachydakis A, Koutroumanis P, Geyushi B, Hanna L. Primary Hyperparathyroidism in Pregnancy Presenting as Intractable Hyperemesis Complicating Psychogenic Anorexia: A Case Report. *J Reprod Med.* 2008;53(9):714–716.

11. Nilsson IL, Adner N, Reihnér E, Palme-Kilander C, Edstrom G, Degerblad M. Primary Hyperparathyroidism in Pregnancy: A Diagnostic and Therapeutic Challenge. *J Womens Health (Larchmt).* 2010;19(6):1117–1121.

6b

Osteoporosis and vitamin D deficiency

FIONA J COOK

KEY POINTS

- Pregnancy and lactation-associated osteoporosis (PLO) is rare but likely underdiagnosed. It is more common in women with underlying risks for bone fragility.
- Clinical presentations of PLO include fragility fractures, which are most commonly vertebral, or transient osteoporosis of the hip, a focal problem unrelated to calcium metabolism or systemic bone resorption.
- The maternal skeleton becomes more vulnerable to fracture due to increase in bone resorption. The bone loss is recovered in most cases by 6–12 months after weaning.
- Treatment approach includes management of any identified reversible secondary causes for skeletal fragility, provision of adequate calcium and vitamin D, consideration for weaning in patients currently lactating, and pharmacologic therapy in select cases.
- There are no randomized controlled trials to guide pharmacologic therapy in PLO, but there is most clinical experience with bisphosphonates in the postpartum period.

- Vitamin D deficiency has a spectrum of severity and is increasingly prevalent in pregnant patients, with higher risk in those with obesity, darker skin, or less sunlight exposure.
- Vitamin D plays an important role in provision of calcium for the fetal skeleton but likely has other roles during pregnancy including immune response regulation.
- Vitamin D deficiency is associated with maternal and fetal complications including preeclampsia, gestational diabetes, preterm delivery, and impaired fetal bone development and growth.
- Screening for vitamin D deficiency in pregnancy should be considered, especially in patients with risk factors.
- Routine vitamin D supplementation of at least 1400 IU daily is recommended to meet increased maternal requirement during pregnancy and lactation.
- Breast milk contains little vitamin D, so breastfed infants require sufficient sunlight exposure or vitamin D supplementation to meet their requirement of 400 IU daily.

PREGNANCY AND LACTATION-ASSOCIATED OSTEOPOROSIS

Epidemiology

- Pregnancy-associated fractures were first described by Fuller Albright in 1948 and postpregnancy osteoporosis was first proposed as a syndrome in 1955.[1,2]
- In a 1985 review, the prevalence of osteoporosis in pregnancy was estimated at 4–8 per million, but the actual prevalence is unclear due to underreporting and underdiagnosis in the case of vertebral fractures (VFs), which may

DOI: 10.1201/9781003027577-36

Table 6b.1 Risk factors leading to low bone mineral density or skeletal fragility

Endocrine	Primary hyperparathyroidism
	Hyperthyroidism
	Hypothalamic or pituitary amenorrhea
	Premature ovarian insufficiency
	Cushing's syndrome
Nutritional	Calcium/vitamin D deficiency
Physical	Small frame
	Low body weight/BMI
Drugs	GnRH analogs
	Depot medroxyprogesterone
	Glucocorticoids
	Proton pump inhibitors
	Anti-epileptics (phenytoin, carbamazepine)
	Cancer chemotherapy
Gastrointestinal	Malabsorptive disorders: Celiac disease, Crohn's disease, cystic fibrosis, bariatric surgery
Renal	Renal calcium leak
	Chronic renal insufficiency
	Renal tubular acidosis
Genetic	Osteogenesis imperfecta
	LRP5 inactivating mutations
	Ehlers-Danlos syndrome
Lifestyle	Tobacco abuse
	Alcohol abuse

be asymptomatic or cause only moderate back pain dismissed as a typical symptom of late pregnancy.[3–5]

- Pregnancy and lactation-associated osteoporosis (PLO) occurs more often in women with risk factors leading to low bone mineral density (BMD) or skeletal fragility prepregnancy (Table 6b.1).[4–7]

- In general, parity and lactation have been found to be neutral or protective regarding a woman's lifetime risk of osteoporotic fracture.[4] However, long-term data on subsequent fracture risk in women with PLO is limited. A prospective cohort study of patients with PLO (secondary causes of osteoporosis excluded) with a median follow-up of 6 years indicated that 24.3% had a subsequent fragility fracture. The same study observed that a greater number of VFs at diagnosis of PLO may correlate with subsequent fracture risk.[5]

Pathophysiology

PREGNANCY

- The fetal skeleton accrues 30 g of calcium by term, 80% of which is acquired during the third trimester.[4,5] The fetal serum calcium exceeds maternal serum calcium due to calcium-binding proteins in the placenta, which transfers calcium against the concentration gradient.[8]

- Starting at 12 weeks gestation, maternal efficiency of calcium absorption doubles, leading to a positive maternal calcium balance by mid-pregnancy.[4] The increase in calcium absorption is partially explained by an increase in calcitriol production, especially in the third trimester.[4,8]

- Modest bone resorption may occur during a normal pregnancy, presumably due to an increase in parathyroid hormone-related

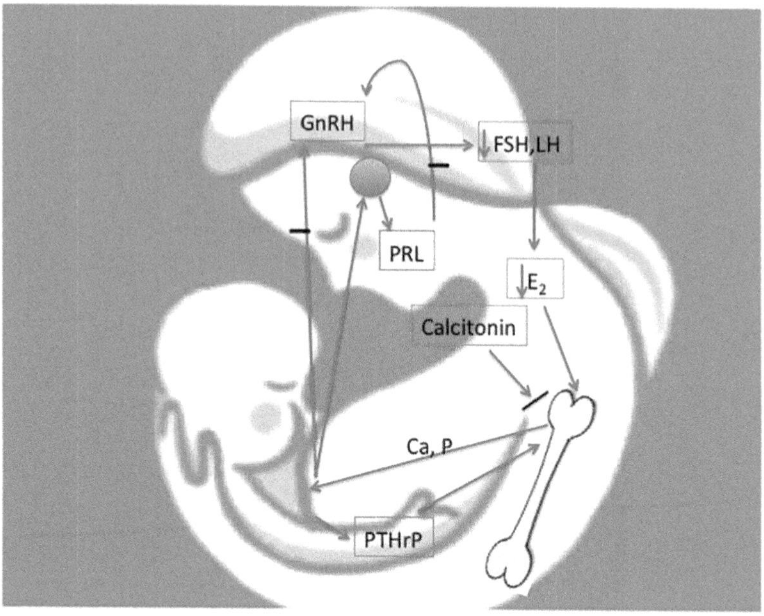

Figure 6b.1 Breast-brain-bone circuit

peptide (PTHrP) production by the placenta and breasts.[4]

- Parathyroid hormone (PTH) tends to be low during pregnancy unless there is inadequate maternal intake of calcium.[4]
- Some studies indicate a small loss of BMD during pregnancy, primarily at trabecular-rich sites.[4,6] The predominance of VFs is attributed to loss of trabecular bone along with the mechanical effects of pregnancy on the spine (weight gain and lumbar lordosis).[5-7]

LACTATION

- To meet a neonate's needs, the average daily maternal calcium loss in milk is approximately 210 mg. Six months of full-time breastfeeding requires four times the mineral delivery of pregnancy.[4,5]
- During lactation, calcium absorption and calcitriol decrease to normal levels and PTH is suppressed, but bone resorption significantly increases in order to provide the needed calcium in milk.[4,5,9]
- Increased resorption is partly due to a decrease in estradiol, which results in receptor activator of nuclear factor kappa (RANK)-mediated increase in osteoclast function.[4,5,7,8]

- The "brain-breast-bone circuit" during lactation appears to be independent of dietary calcium intake (Figure 6b.1).[4,9]
  - PTH-related peptide (PTHrP) secreted by the breast in response to suckling also increases bone resorption and enhances reabsorption of calcium in the kidney tubules.[4,5,7,8]
  - BMD decreases by 1–3% per month in the first 6 months of lactation, primarily at trabecular sites.[4,9] The decline in BMD correlates with the amount of milk produced.[9]
  - Circulating calcitonin counters by inhibiting osteoclastic bone resorption to protect the maternal skeleton from excessive bone loss.[4,9]
  - Bone lost during lactation is generally recovered within 6–12 months after weaning, likely mediated by the subsequent decrease in PTHrP and rise in estradiol, along with an increase in PTH and calcitriol.[4,5,9]

TRANSIENT OSTEOPOROSIS OF THE HIP

- Transient osteoporosis of the hip, also known as reflex sympathetic dystrophy or complex regional pain syndrome type 1, occurs in the third trimester or early postpartum.[4,6] The patient presents with a limp, hip pain, or a hip fracture.

- Osteopenia of the femoral head and neck is seen on plain radiographs and dual-energy X-ray absorptiometry (DXA) and edema of the femoral head and marrow is seen on magnetic resonance imaging (MRI).
- The etiology is unclear, but proposed theories include pressure on the femoral vein or obturator nerve by the pregnant uterus.[4]

Diagnosis

- There are no uniform diagnostic criteria for PLO.[7]
- The most common presentation is with spontaneous, often multiple, VFs in late pregnancy or during lactation up to 18 months postpartum.[4,7] Most patients present early postpartum with back pain.[7]
- Typically, bone resorption markers will be increased and BMD Z-scores, particularly in the spine, will be low.[4,5,7]
- If postpartum, plain radiographs of the spine and/or hip and BMD with DXA should be obtained. MRI of an affected hip will confirm the diagnosis of transient osteoporosis of the hip.[4]
- Laboratory investigation for underlying contributing factors is similar to that in nonpregnant women with premature osteoporosis (Table 6b.2).[4]

Treatment

- Any reversible contributors to bone loss should be addressed if possible.[4]
- Calcium and vitamin D nutrition should be ensured such that the total daily calcium intake is at least 1200 mg and the vitamin D level is maintained at 30 ng/mL or higher.[4,10]
- Avoidance of heavy lifting but maintenance of mobility is important. Short-term corset support of the spine may be considered.[4]
- For fractures during lactation, weaning is advised.[5]
- Pharmacologic therapy should be delayed in most cases for 12–18 months until the extent of spontaneous recovery is known.[4]
- There are no randomized clinical trials of any pharmacologic therapies for PLO.

Table 6b.2 Laboratory investigation for pregnancy and lactation-associated osteoporosis

	Laboratory evaluation
Hematology	Complete blood count (CBC)
	SPEP[a]
	Ferritin or iron[a]
Biochemistry	Electrolytes
	eGFR
	Albumin-corrected serum calcium
	Phosphate
	Alkaline phosphatase
	Bone turnover markers[a]
	24-hr urine calcium[a]
Endocrine	25-OH vitamin D
	Intact PTH
	TSH
	PTHrP[a]
	24-hr urine free cortisol or late-night salivary cortisol[a]

[a] If clinically indicated

- Bisphosphonates cross the placenta and could interfere with fetal bone development, even in a future pregnancy due to their long half-life in bone.[4,6,7]
  - A prospective study of 12 postpartum patients treated with weaning along with alendronate or zoledronic acid and calcium and vitamin D supplementation indicated a decrease in bone turnover markers and an increase in BMD, but there was a lack of placebo control so it is unclear if bisphosphonates were better than spontaneous recovery.[7]
  - In a summary of BP studies for PLO, BMD increases ranged from 5% to 28.3% at the spine, 2.6–6.5% at the femoral neck, and 1.1–8% at the hip sites after 1 year of treatment.[7]
  - A literature review of 78 cases of bisphosphonate use during pregnancy found no obvious problems in the majority but noted transient hypocalcemia in infancy in three cases, talipes equinovarus in one case, and nonskeletal malformations in two cases.[11]
- In available studies, use of teriparatide in PLO has resulted in significant BMD increases at the total hip after one year of treatment.[7] However, lifetime use of teriparatide should be limited

to 2 years in most cases so it may be prudent to save this therapy for older age. Also, teriparatide use is contraindicated if the epiphyses of the mother are open.[4]

- Denosumab crosses the placenta and causes an osteopetrotic phenotype in monkeys in utero.[4] A few cases of denosumab therapy for postpartum PLO have been reported with resultant increase in trabecular volume and thickness of the radius and tibia but delaying conception for 6 months after the last dose was suggested.[7]
- The effect of vertebro- or kyphoplasty is unclear but there is evidence that mechanical strain will be induced on adjacent vertebrae.
- Transient osteoporosis of the hip is self-limited, but if fracture occurs, surgery may be necessary. Women should be advised that this condition may recur with subsequent pregnancies.[4]

DEFICIENCY OF VITAMIN D IN PREGNANCY AND LACTATION

Epidemiology

- Vitamin D deficiency is a growing health concern worldwide, largely due to decreased exposure to sunlight.[8] Populations at risk include those living at altitudes with less sunlight, darker-skinned races, and obese people.[10,12–14] Obese adults (BMI ≥ 30 kg/m²) are at high risk for vitamin D deficiency because the body fat sequesters the fat-soluble vitamin.[14]
- The increased prevalence of vitamin D deficiency during pregnancy raises concern regarding associated adverse outcomes. There are numerous studies on this topic, but results are inconsistent, largely due to variations in study population and design. It remains unclear as to whether vitamin D deficiency is a contributing cause for certain pregnancy complications or an associated marker.[8] The increased prevalence of vitamin D deficiency in obese women who have a higher prevalence of gestational diabetes makes analysis of cause and effect more complex.[10]

Pathophysiology

- The most important role of vitamin D in pregnancy is to increase maternal calcium absorption and placental calcium transport to adapt to the needs of bone mineral accrual by the fetus in the third trimester.[8]
- Under stable circumstances, the serum 25-hydroxy vitamin D (25OHD) concentration is relatively constant throughout pregnancy, but serum 1,25-dihydroxy vitamin D (calcitriol) increases by 2–3 times due to increased placental and renal 1-α hydroxylase activity, vitamin D-binding proteins, and placental vitamin D receptors.[10,13]
- 25OHD crosses the placenta and is the main source of vitamin D for the fetus.[7,10] The fetal kidney expresses 1-α hydroxylase.[8]
- Vitamin D has other roles including immune regulation, anti-inflammation, and release of the antimicrobial peptide cathelicidin from the placenta.[8,13]
- Calcitriol acts on the placenta to stimulate endometrial decidualization, control synthesis of estradiol and progesterone, and regulate human chorionic gonadotropin (hCG) and human placental lactogen (hPL) expression.
- Vitamin D also enhances maternal tolerance to prenatal and fetal alloantigens.[8]
- Effect on maternal and fetal outcomes:
  - Many studies suggest an association between vitamin D deficiency and preeclampsia, theoretically through the role of vitamin D in immune homeostasis, angiogenesis, and the health of vascular smooth muscle and endothelium.[8] A meta-analysis indicated that women supplemented with vitamin D had a lower risk of preeclampsia of borderline significance, but women supplemented with both vitamin D and calcium had a significantly lower risk.[15]
  - Gestational diabetes and preterm delivery have been associated with vitamin D deficiency and supplementation should be considered to reduce these complications, based on limited available evidence.[8,10]
  - Cesarean section, recurrent pregnancy loss, bacterial vaginosis, and postpartum depression have been studied in association with vitamin D deficiency with conflicting results.[8,10]
  - Maternal vitamin D deficiency is associated with impaired bone development and fetal growth. Most studies suggest that supplementation during pregnancy has a

positive impact on fetal anthropometry but not birth weight.

- Due to the involvement of vitamin D in immune regulation, the role of maternal vitamin D deficiency in offspring respiratory infections, allergies, and autism has been studied without definitive conclusions.[8]

Diagnosis

- Maternal vitamin D depletion covers a continuum of severity.[12]
- Vitamin D deficiency is defined by serum 25OHD <20 ng/mL and insufficiency by serum 25OHD 20–30 ng/mL.[8,14] The normal range for serum 25OHD is the same in pregnant and nonpregnant women.
- Severe vitamin D deficiency is characterized by intestinal calcium and phosphorus malabsorption, hypocalcemia, secondary hyperparathyroidism, and demineralization of bone (osteomalacia), while vitamin D insufficiency may induce mild hyperparathyroidism and gradual bone loss.[12]
- Endocrine Society guidelines recommend that large groups of the normal population undergo screening, including patients with African American or Hispanic ethnicity, obese people, and pregnant women.[14] However, this is controversial as the cost may be difficult to justify. Screening should certainly be performed in pregnant women at increased risk for vitamin D deficiency due to a chronic medical condition such as intestinal malabsorption (including bariatric surgery), liver or kidney disease, or use of drugs such as corticosteroids, anticonvulsants, antifungals, or HIV medications.[12]

Treatment

- Vitamin D requirements are greater in pregnancy.[14,16,17] Endocrine Society guidelines recommend that routine daily supplements during pregnancy and lactation should include a prenatal vitamin containing 400 IU of vitamin D with an additional vitamin D supplement containing at least 1000 IU.[14] A randomized controlled trial showed that 4000 IU of vitamin D_3 daily led to a decrease in pregnancy complications.[18]

- Vitamin D supplements are available as prescriptions or over the counter. As prescriptions, vitamin D_2 (ergocalciferol) is available in capsules that contain 50,000 IU or liquid which contains 8000 IU/mL. Vitamin D_3 (cholecalciferol) in multiple doses is available over the counter.[10]
- The goal level of 25OHD during pregnancy and lactation is a minimum of 30 ng/mL per Endocrine Society guidelines or 20 ng/mL per the Institute of Medicine, with higher levels probably advantageous, depending on the population.[14,16]
- Human milk contains low amounts of vitamin D, even in the setting of maternal vitamin D sufficiency. To satisfy the requirements of an infant who is fed only breast milk, the mother requires 4000 to 6000 IU/day to transfer enough vitamin D into her milk. Alternatively, the breastfed infant may be supplemented with 400 IU daily.[14]
- For nonpregnant adults with vitamin D deficiency, recommended treatment is 50,000 IU D_2 or D_3 weekly or 6000 IU of D_2 or D_3 daily for 8 weeks to achieve a 25OHD level above 30 ng/mL, followed by maintenance therapy of 1500–2000 IU daily.[14] There is no evidence to suggest any different strategy in a pregnant or lactating woman.
- Concomitant calcium supplements should be provided if needed to ensure a total daily calcium intake of at least 1200 mg.[4]

REFERENCES

1. Albright F, Reifenstein EC. Parathyroid Glands and Metabolic Bone Disease. Williams & Wilkins, Baltimore, 1948.
2. Nordin BE, Roper A. Post-pregnancy osteoporosis; a syndrome? Lancet 1955;268:431–434.
3. Smith R, Stevenson JC, Winearls CG et al. Osteoporosis of pregnancy. Lancet 1985;1(8439):1178–1180.
4. Kovacs CS, Ralston SH. Presentation and management of osteoporosis in association with pregnancy and lactation. Osteoporos Int. 2015; 26:2223–2241.
5. Kyvernitakis I, Reuter TC, Hellmeyer L et al. Subsequent fracture risk of women with pregnancy and lactation-associated

osteoporosis after a median of 6 years of follow-up. Osteoporos Int. 2018;29: 135–142.

6. Hardcastle SA, Yahya F, Bhalla AK. Pregnancy-associated osteoporosis: A UK case series and literature review. Osteoporos Int. 2019;30:939–948.

7. Li L, Zhang J, Gao P et al. Clinical characteristics and bisphosphonates treatment of rare pregnancy- and lactation-associated osteoporosis. Clin Rheumatol. 2018;37:3141–3150.

8. Agarwal S, Kovilam O, Agrawak DK. Vitamin D and its impact on maternal and fetal outcomes in pregnancy: A critical review. Crit Rev Food Sci Nutr. 2018;58(5):755–769.

9. Wysolmerski JJ. Interactions between breast, bone, and brain regulate mineral and skeletal metabolism during lactation. Ann N Y Acad Sci. 2010;1192:161–169.

10. Dovnik A, Mujezinovic F. The association of vitamin D levels with common pregnancy complications. Nutrients. 2018;10:867.

11. Stathopoulos IP, Liakou CG, Katsalira A et al. The use of bisphosphonates in women prior to or during pregnancy and lactation. Hormones 2011;10(4):280–291.

12. Gallagher, JC. Vitamin D Deficiency and Insufficiency. In: Rosen, CJ, editor. Primer on the Metabolic Bone Diseases and Disorders of Mineral Metabolism. 8th ed. Oxford: Wiley and Blackwell; 2013. p. 624–663.

13. Karras, SN, Wagner CL, Castracane VD. Understanding vitamin D metabolism in pregnancy: From physiology to pathophysiology and clinical outcomes. Metabolism 2018;86:112–123.

14. Holick MF, Binkley NC, Bischoff-Ferrari HA et al. Evaluation, treatment, and prevention of vitamin D deficiency: An Endocrine Society Clinical Practice Guideline. J Clin Endocrinol Metab 2011;96:1911–1930.

15. De-Regil LM, Palacios C, Lombardo LK, Peña-Rosas JP. Vitamin D supplementation for women during pregnancy. Cochrane Database Syst Rev. 2016;1(1):CD008873.

16. Mithal A, Kalra S. Vitamin D supplementation in pregnancy. Indian J Endocrinol Metab. 2014;18(5):593–596.

17. Hollis, BW, Wagner, CL. Vitamin D and pregnancy: Skeletal effects, nonskeletal effects, and birth outcomes. Calcif Tissue Int. 2013;92:128–139.

18. Hollis BW, Wagner CL. Vitamin D requirements during lactation: High-dose maternal supplementation as therapy to prevent hypovitaminosis D for both the mother and the nursing infant. Am J Clin Nutr. 2004;80:1752S–1758S.

CHAPTER 7

Special Considerations

Transgender health in pregnancy and the postpartum period

JESSICA PERINI

KEY POINTS

- Fertility can be impaired in patients using gender-affirming hormones.
- For transgender men with intact reproductive organs, fertility can be accomplished and pregnancy carried to term.
- Testosterone should be discontinued prior to conception and not resumed until after delivery.

- Pregnancy in transgender men can lead to significant worsening of gender dysphoria.
- Healthcare providers must proactively prepare and educate their office and workplace colleagues regarding use of gender-inclusive and affirming language and provision of patient-centered care.

EPIDEMIOLOGY

- Transgender men are individuals who were assigned female sex at birth but who identify as male.
- As few as 8% of transgender men have had a hysterectomy.[1] Therefore, the majority of transgender men have retained their female reproductive organs and thus their potential for pregnancy.
- In one report of a cohort of pregnant transgender men, 20% had become pregnant while using testosterone and while amenorrheic.[2]
- Up to 50% or more of transgender pregnant men do not seek prenatal care.[2]
- No significant differences have been noted in pregnancy, delivery, or birth outcomes between transgender men who had used testosterone prior to pregnancy and those who had not.[2]

- Guidelines are lacking regarding best practice in providing gender-affirming and patient-centered care for transgender men seeking pre-, peri-, or postnatal care.

PATHOPHYSIOLOGY

- An inherent desired effect of gender-affirming hormone therapy (GAHT) in transgender men is suppression of endogenous estrogen.
- Exogenous testosterone use typically leads to anovulation and amenorrhea, a commonly desired outcome for transgender men. Fertility is therefore impaired due to suppression of the hypothalamic-pituitary-ovarian axis.
- Testosterone use may also increase insulin resistance, a metabolic abnormality associated with anovulatory cycles and impaired fertility.[3,4]

DOI: 10.1201/9781003027577-38

- Discontinuation of testosterone may or may not lead to resumption of ovulation. While GAHT can impair fertility, discontinuation of GAHT may result in return of menstrual cycles and conception ability.[5,6] In one report, 80% of transgender men experienced menstrual cycle resumption within 6 months of testosterone discontinuation.[2]
- In transgender men who have had suppression of ovulation since adolescence, there is no clear data to indicate when or whether spontaneous ovulation will resume after cessation of GAHT.
- There is no definitive information regarding efficacy of ovulation induction in this population.[6]
- Pregnancy remains a possibility if the patient has functional uterus, vagina, and ovaries.[7]
- Psychosocial aspects of pregnancy often present the biggest challenges for transgender men during pregnancy.
  - Gender dysphoria can worsen during pregnancy due to physical changes such as enlarging breast tissue.[8]
  - Public attitudes toward pregnant men can create uncomfortable environments.
  - Medical care services themselves may present patients with a hostile environment leading to a decrease in access to or utilization of prenatal care.[9] One study noted that only half of transgender men received physician-led prenatal care.[2]

TREATMENT

- Future reproductive plans should be discussed with all transgender patients. If interested in future fertility, referral to reproductive endocrinology is important for discussion of fertility preservation options prior to initiation of GAHT.[10]
- Patients who do not wish to become pregnant should be advised that GAHT is not a reliable form of contraception and additional forms of contraception should be utilized.[2]
- Testosterone discontinuation
  - In patients who are amenorrheic on current GAHT, cessation of testosterone may help hypothalamic-pituitary-gonadal axis recovery and stimulate resumption of ovulation.

- Testosterone (pregnancy category X) use is contraindicated in pregnancy due to androgenic and teratogenic effects on the fetus. Therefore, testosterone should be discontinued, preferably if attempting conception or upon recognition of pregnancy.
- There is no recommended time interval between cessation of testosterone and conception.
- Discontinuation of gender-affirming hormones may lead to significant gender dysphoria.
- For patients actively planning pregnancy, other options for fertility include using the patient's own or donor oocytes and sperm from a spouse, partner, or donor.
- Medical and technological assistance to enhance fertility can be considered.
  - In one study, 7% of transgender men required fertility medications to become pregnant and 12% required assisted reproductive technology including artificial insemination, in vitro fertilization, or gamete intrafallopian transfer.[2]
  - Uterine transplant has been successful in cisgender women but, to date, no successful cases have been reported in transgender men. This may become an option in the future for transgender men who have previously undergone gender-affirming hysterectomy.
  - Ectopic implantation of an embryo is not recommended due to significant risks to both fetus and the pregnant patient.[11]
- Psychosocial aspects of care
  - All patients with gender dysphoria are advised to have a mental health provider (MHP) work with them during the transition process. For many who have transitioned, however, frequency of contact with a MHP may have diminished. Patients should be encouraged to accept referral to an appropriate MHP as they progress through pregnancy and experience a decline in gender-affirming hormone levels.
  - All providers who provide care to transgender patients should counsel front desk staff, nurses, and the labor and delivery team in preparation for medical and social

aspects involved in caring for transgender pregnant patients.

- Healthcare providers should advise use of gender-neutral language by all who interact with patients, including sonographers, to discourage discrimination and provide affirming and inclusive language.
- Patients should be asked whether they prefer to be referred to as father, mother, or other during the pregnancy.

- At second trimester and later in the pregnancy, providers should review the patient's plan for future fertility, resumption of GAHT, and contraceptive options.
- Postnatal care and lactation
  - Providers should discuss preferred breast-feeding terminology with patients (e.g., breastfeeding, chestfeeding, nursing, or another term expressed by the patient).[12]
  - Patients who have undergone gender-affirming top surgery may be able to chestfeed but may have to supplement with formula. If there is no history of gender-affirming mastectomy, chestfeeding is expected to be possible.
  - Breast binding can slow or inhibit milk supply by mammary glands and ductal tissue. It can, however, increase the risk of duct blockage and mastitis.
  - Patients may consider use of donor milk.
  - Testosterone therapy is not recommended while nursing; however, one study showed that testosterone from pellet implants was not measurably excreted into breast milk.[13]

REFERENCES

1. Hahn M, Sheran N, Weber S, Cohan D, Obedin-Maliver J. Providing patient-centered perinatal care for transgender men and gender-diverse individuals: A collaborative multidisciplinary team approach. *Obstet Gynecol.* 2019;134(5):959–963.
2. Light AD, Obedin-Maliver J, Sevelius JM, Kerns JL. Transgender men who experienced pregnancy after female-to-male gender transitioning. *Obstet Gynecol.* 2014;124(6):1120–1127.
3. Matsui S, Yasui T, Tani A et al. Associations of estrogen and testosterone with insulin resistance in pre- and postmenopausal women with and without hormone therapy. *Int J Endocrinol Metab.* 2013;11(2):65–70.
4. Fica S, Albu A, Constantin M, Dobri GA. Insulin resistance and fertility in polycystic ovary syndrome. *J Med Life.* 2008;1(4):415–422.
5. Cheng PJ, Pastuszak AW, Myers JB, Goodwin IA, Hotaling JM. Fertility concerns of the transgender patient. *Transl Androl Urol.* 2019;8(3):209–218.
6. Steinle K. Hormonal management of the female-to-male transgender patient. *J Midwifery Womens Health.* 2011;56(3):293–302.
7. Obedin-Maliver J, Makadon HJ. Transgender men and pregnancy. *Obstet Med.* 2016;9(1): 4–8. doi:10.1177/1753495X15612658.
8. Dutton L, Koenig K, Fennie K. Gynecologic care of the female-to-male transgender man. *J Midwifery Womens Health.* 2008; 53(4):331–337.
9. Beatie T. Labor of love. *Advocate.* March 2008. https://www.advocate.com/news/2008/03/26/labor-love
10. Hembree WC, Cohen-Kettenis PT, Gooren L et al. Endocrine treatment of gender-dysphoric/gender-incongruent persons: An Endocrine Society Clinical Practice Guideline [published correction appears in *J Clin Endocrinol Metab.* 2018 Feb 1;103(2):699] [published correction appears in *J Clin Endocrinol Metab.* 2018 Jul 1;103(7):2758–2759]. *J Clin Endocrinol Metab.* 2017;102(11):3869–3903.
11. Leith W. Pregnant men: Hard to stomach? *The Telegraph*, London. April 2008. https://www.telegraph.co.uk/men/active/mens-health/3354220/Pregnant-men-hard-to-stomach.html
12. MacDonald T, Noel-Weiss J, West D et al. Transmasculine individuals' experiences with lactation, chestfeeding, and gender identity: A qualitative study. *BMC Pregnancy Childbirth.* 2016;16:106. Published 2016 May 16.
13. Glaser RL, Newman M, Parsons M, Zava D, Glaser-Garbrick D. Safety of maternal testosterone therapy during breast feeding. *Int J Pharm Compd.* 2009;13(4):314–317.

Endocrine tumors in pregnancy

VALERIE B GALVAN TURNER

KEY POINTS

- Gestational trophoblastic disease (GTD) refers to interrelated tumors arising from the placental villous trophoblastic tissue.[1] The term includes benign hydatidiform molar pregnancies (complete and partial) as well as malignant conditions (invasive mole, choriocarcinoma, placental site trophoblastic tumor). These malignant conditions are then termed gestational trophoblastic neoplasia (GTN).
- Symptoms that raise suspicion for molar pregnancies include vaginal bleeding, uterine size out of proportion to gestational dating, and significantly elevated human chorionic gonadotropin (hCG) levels.
- Evacuation of pregnancy is key in treatment of GTD followed by serial hCG surveillance.
- Choriocarcinoma is a rare and aggressive malignancy that falls within the subtypes of GTD. It typically develops in patients with a known history of molar pregnancy.
- The mainstay of treatment of choriocarcinoma includes chemotherapy +/– surgical intervention.

MOLAR PREGNANCY

Epidemiology

- The prevalence of molar pregnancies is based on multiple risk factors, which include extremes of maternal age (greatest risk with age >40 years) and history of prior hydatidiform mole. The risk of a second molar pregnancy is 1–2%, with further increased risk of third molar pregnancy at 25%.[2] Additional risk factors include geography, dietary factors, poor nutritional status, and socioeconomic status.[3]
- Incidence of complete molar pregnancy in the United States is 1:1000 to 1:1500.[1,2] Within the United States, Native American women living in New Mexico are the highest risk population for GTD.[3,4]
- With inclusion of the whole of North America, South America, and Europe, the incidence of GTD increases to 1:500 to 1:1000 pregnancies. The incidence is higher still in East Asia, approaching 1:120 pregnancies.[3]
- Incidence of partial molar pregnancy, however, is unknown.[5] This is likely due to underdiagnosis secondary to lack of histology and karyotype analysis with spontaneous miscarriages and induced abortions.

Pathophysiology

COMPLETE HYDATIDIFORM MOLE

- A complete hydatidiform mole is a result of a paternal homologous chromosome pattern. This occurs when a single sperm (90%) or dispermy (10%) fertilizes an egg with absent

DOI: 10.1201/9781003027577-39

Table 7b.1 Characteristics of molar pregnancies

Characteristics	Complete mole	Partial mole
Karyotype (most common)	Diploid (46XX)	Triploid (69XXY)
Origin	Paternal	Maternal and paternal
Fetal tissue/amnion	Absent	Present
Hydropic villi	Pronounced/generalized	Variable/focal
Trophoblastic proliferation	Variable/marked	Focal
Malignant sequelae	6–36%	<5%

nuclear DNA.[1,2] The most common resulting karyotype is 46XX (85%) and less likely 46XY.[6]

- The result is extensive trophoblastic proliferation and edema of villous stroma. All chorionic villi are avascular and vesicular. In addition, there are no amniotic membranes and no fetal tissue (see Table 7b.1).[7]

PARTIAL HYDATIDIFORM MOLE

- The majority of partial molar pregnancies contain a triploid karyotype. This occurs when an egg is fertilized by multiple sperm with a resulting 69XXY or 69XXX (or rare 69XYY) karyotype.
- The result is focal and mild hyperplasia of trophoblastic elements and a mixture of normal and hydropic chorionic villi. Amniotic membranes and fetal tissue are both present. However, given the triploid nature, fetal development is typically severely hindered by congenital anomalies and is often nonviable (see Table 7b.1).[5,6,8]

Diagnosis

- Vaginal bleeding is the most common presenting symptom of hydatidiform molar pregnancies. Other initial presenting symptoms include physical exam findings indicating uterine size exceeding gestational date and significantly elevated hCG levels typically exceeding 100,000 mIU/mL.[1]
- Ultrasound imaging is key in the diagnosis of hydatidiform molar pregnancies.
  - With routine availability and improvement of ultrasound technology, molar pregnancies are now diagnosed more frequently in the early first trimester.

- Due to the trophoblastic proliferation and vesicular nature of chorionic villi, a complete molar pregnancy has a characteristic "snowstorm" appearance.
- Other ultrasound findings include a uniform multicystic endometrial cavity pattern with diffuse echolucent and echodense structures containing grape-like vesicles.[1,7]
- Because fetal tissue is present, partial molar pregnancies are more difficult to diagnose but fetal anomalies related to trisomy nature are common.[7,8]
- Once diagnosis is made, evaluation for additional medical complications related to GTD is important, including preeclampsia, hyperemesis and resulting electrolyte disturbances, anemia, and hyperthyroidism.[1,9] In addition, the presence of bilateral adnexal masses secondary to theca luteal cysts further contributes to elevated hCG levels with similar physiology to ovarian hyperstimulation. The enlarged ovaries can lead to significant abdominal discomfort, torsion, and rarely, infarction or hemorrhage.[6,7]
- Due to the risk of GTN, chest X-ray is recommended for evaluation of metastasis. Given the array of possible medical comorbidities associated with molar pregnancies, further workup following diagnosis of GTD should include[1,9]:
  - Serum hCG level
  - Pelvic ultrasound
  - Complete blood count (CBC) with differential
  - Type and screen
  - Thyroid studies
  - Serum chemistry panel
  - Renal and liver studies
  - Chest X-ray

Treatment

- Evacuation of pregnancy is key to treatment.
  - Determining route of evacuation is dependent on the patient's fertility plans but is most commonly performed via suction curettage under ultrasound guidance for completeness, particularly if uterine size is >14 weeks gestation.
  - Hysterectomy can be considered as safe evacuation if future fertility is undesired, particularly in women of advanced maternal age, given increased risk of GTN in patients over age 40 (54%).
  - Medical induction of labor and hysterotomy is not supported and strongly discouraged as means of evacuation.[1,8,9]
- Given the structural similarity of hCG to thyroid-stimulating hormone (TSH), thyroid storm is possible at the time of evacuation and surgical management if significantly elevated hCG levels (>500,000 mIU/mL) are present or if there is evidence of preexisting hyperthyroidism.
- Consultation and communication with the anesthesiology team are critical as β-adrenergic blocker administration at time of anesthesia induction is recommended.
- Potential intraoperative complications include[9]:
  - Hemorrhage
  - Respiratory distress secondary to fluid replacement
  - Trophoblastic pulmonary embolization
  - Preeclampsia
  - High-output heart failure secondary to thyroid storm
- Oxytocin uterotonic use for post-evacuation bleeding control should not be administered until in the operating room to decrease risk of embolization of trophoblastic tissue.[2] It is recommended that oxytocin be administered at the time of suction curettage and immediately post-procedure.
- Immediately following evacuation, Rho (D) immunoglobulin should be administered for Rh-negative patients.[1,8,9] This is not necessary if hysterectomy is performed.
- Whether evacuation of pregnancy with aspiration or hysterectomy is performed, close surveillance with serial hCG monitoring is important.
  - Serum hCG levels should be checked weekly until less than the reference range for 3 consecutive weeks.
  - Following normalization of hCG levels for three consecutive weeks, monitoring should then proceed to monthly surveillance of serum hCG levels for a minimum of six months to ensure no progression to gestational trophoblastic neoplasia (GTN).[1,2,8,9]
- Hysterectomy by itself does not eliminate the chance of GTN development. During the minimum 6-month surveillance period, reliable contraception is critical to avoid confusing a new pregnancy with progression to GTN.
- Prophylactic chemotherapy with methotrexate or dactinomycin at the time of pregnancy evacuation is not recommended or shown to decrease progression to GTN in low-risk patients.[5] Prophylactic chemotherapy should only be considered in high-risk patients and in patients for whom adequate hCG monitoring cannot be performed.[1]

POST-MOLAR GTN

- During the minimum 6-month surveillance period, concern for malignant progression to GTN rises with any of the following[10]:
  - Rising or plateaued serum hCG values; if this occurs from one week to the next, weekly surveillance should continue instead of deescalating to a monthly monitoring
  - hCG plateau for four consecutive values for ≥3 weeks
  - hCG rise ≥10% for three values for ≥2 weeks
  - hCG values >20,000 mIU/mL at 4 weeks post initial surgical evacuation
  - Persistently elevated hCG levels >5 mIU/mL after 6-month surveillance, even if a continuous decline has occurred
  - Persistent or heavy vaginal bleeding
  - Any evidence of metastatic disease; metastases can arise in the lung (most common site with imaging demonstrating a lung

opacity >2 cm), brain, liver, or gastrointestinal tract

- Any intraabdominal or gastrointestinal bleeding

- After confirmation of a GTN diagnosis with any of the above criteria, the patient should be evaluated by a professional who specializes in GTN, such as a gynecologist-oncologist. In addition, further workup should include[10]:
  - Repeat CBC with differential
  - Repeat serum hCG
  - Repeat chemistry profile
  - Repeat liver, renal, and thyroid studies
  - Repeat imaging:
    - Chest/abdominal/pelvic CT scan with IV contrast
    - MRI (preferred) or CT brain with contrast if pulmonary metastases are present
    - Pelvic ultrasound or MRI

- An increase in both total and hyperglycosylated hCG is associated with cytotrophoblastic invasion. This can help differentiate GTN from quiescent gestational trophoblastic disease (GTD), which is not associated with hyperglycosylated hCG.

- At least six major variants of hCG can be detected in the serum and most institutions utilize a rapid, automated radiolabeled monoclonal antibody sandwich assay to measure the various mixtures of hCG molecules. If there is clinical suspicion of a false positive test, phantom hCG should be ruled out by testing urine hCG, serial dilution of serum, or sending the serum and urine to an hCG reference laboratory. The clinician should also rule out hCG α-subunit cross-reactivity with luteinizing hormone (LH) produced by the pituitary which, if elevated, can lead to falsely elevated hCG levels.[1]

CHORIOCARCINOMA

Epidemiology

- The incidence of choriocarcinoma varies worldwide.[1,11] Data indicates an increased risk in women with Asian, Native American, and African American backgrounds.[1,12]

- In Europe and North America, about 1/40,000 pregnant patients and 1/40 patients with hydatidiform moles develop choriocarcinoma. These incidences are significantly higher in Southeast Asia and Japan, with development of choriocarcinoma in 9.2/40,000 pregnant women and 3.3/40 patients with hydatidiform moles. Higher still, in China, it is estimated that 1/2882 pregnant women will develop choriocarcinoma.[1,11]

- Nongestational choriocarcinoma is incredibly rare and comprises <0.1% of ovarian malignancies (germ cell tumors).[13] Like other germ cell tumors, nongestational choriocarcinoma often occurs in children and young adults with some studies citing incidence in prepubescent children of 50%.[12]

Pathophysiology

- Gestational choriocarcinoma develops from abnormal trophoblastic cells, which undergo hyperplasia and anaplasia with resulting malignant transformation. This occurs most frequently following a molar pregnancy, abortion, or normal pregnancy (in order of frequency).[12,14]

- Nongestational choriocarcinoma arises from pluripotent germ cells. Thus, it can affect both females and males, but it is more commonly diagnosed in females.

- Choriocarcinomas spread by blood vessel invasion and exhibit abundant hemorrhage and necrosis on gross examination. On microscopic examination, a plexiform of multinucleated syncytiotrophoblast and cytotrophoblast cells is noted.[14] Syncytiotrophoblast cells produce hCG and are formed from cytotrophoblast cells. Immunohistochemical markers include human placental lactogen (hPL), β-hCG, Ki-67, and sometimes Mel-CAM (CD146).[10]

- The pathogenesis of choriocarcinoma is not fully understood, although studies have shown an overexpression of p53 and MDM2 with no evidence of somatic mutation. High levels of HLA-G (a nonclassic MHC class I molecule) are expressed in choriocarcinoma, which functions to inactivate the local immune system and promote tumor growth. Additionally, choriocarcinomas may derive their invasive and metastatic capabilities from their ability to express increased concentrations of matrix metalloproteinases (MMP) and decreased levels of tissue inhibitors of metalloproteinases (TIMPs).[15]

Diagnosis

- Patients with choriocarcinoma will typically present after a known molar pregnancy after serial hCG monitoring and diagnosis of GTN.
- Choriocarcinoma should be a diagnosis of exclusion, as one should first rule out normal pregnancy or multifetal gestation; however, it should remain in the differential diagnosis in patients presenting with very elevated serum hCG levels.
- Due to elevations in hCG levels, patients can present with abnormal uterine bleeding, gynecomastia (in men and children), or hyperthyroidism.[11,13]
- A thorough history and physical examination should first be performed with focus on the obstetric and social histories with particular attention to the reproductive history, noting any molar pregnancies and abortions or miscarriages that can increase the risk of developing choriocarcinoma.
- A thorough review of systems should be obtained, taking careful note of symptoms that could indicate metastases to common organs such as lungs, liver, gastrointestinal tract, and brain.
- The physical examination should be tailored for evaluation of findings that could indicate the presence of metastatic disease including a pelvic exam.
- If not yet done, evaluation should also include[16]:
  - CBC with differential
  - Coagulation studies
  - Body chemistries
  - Renal and liver function panels
  - Type and screen
  - Quantitative hCG
  - CT of the chest, abdomen, and pelvis (with IV contrast if the patient meets criteria)
  - MRI of the brain, or CT if an MRI cannot be done

Table 7b.2 FIGO staging system for GTN[a]

Stage	Criteria
I	Tumor confined to the uterus
II	Tumor extends to other genital structures (ovary, fallopian tubes, vagina, broad ligaments) by metastasis or direct extension
III	Lung metastasis
IV	All other distant metastases

[a] Adapted from AJCC Cancer Staging Manual, Eighth Edition, 2017.

- Choriocarcinoma is most often diagnosed by elevated hCG levels in conjunction with metastatic disease.

STAGING

- There are four stages of GTN (see Table 7b.2).

Treatment

- For patients with low-risk GTN or gestational choriocarcinoma, the recommended treatment is single-agent systemic chemotherapy with methotrexate or dactinomycin.
- Those with high-risk GTN or gestational or nongestational choriocarcinoma should be treated with multi-agent systemic chemotherapy +/− surgical management as indicated.[12]
- Clinical trials are currently underway to evaluate the effectiveness of immunotherapy for the treatment of refractory disease.
- Radiation has a limited role in the treatment of choriocarcinoma but is often used to limit the complications from hemorrhage from metastatic lesions to the brain and liver.[12]
- Prognosis:
  - If left untreated, choriocarcinoma is highly metastatic and will likely result in death. With the use of chemotherapy, many patients can achieve cure.
  - Low-risk gestational choriocarcinoma has almost 100% survival in women treated with chemotherapy.
  - High-risk gestational choriocarcinoma patients have 91–93% survival when utilizing multi-agent chemotherapy with or without multi-modal treatment.[16]

Table 7b.3 Prognostic scoring index for GTN[a]

Factor	Risk score			
	0	1	2	4
Age (years)	<40	≥40	—	—
Prior pregnancy	Hydatidiform mole	Abortion	Term pregnancy	—
Interval from index pregnancy (months)	<4	4–6	7–12	>12
Pretreatment hCG (IU/L)	$<10^3$	$10^3–10^4$	$10^4–10^5$	$>10^5$
Largest tumor size, including uterus (cm)	<3	3–4	≥5	—
Number of metastatic sites	0	1–4	5–8	>8
Failed chemotherapy	—	—	Single drug	Two or more drugs
Total score[b]	—	—	—	—

[a] Adapted from AJCC Cancer Staging Manual, Eighth Edition, 2017.
[b] The total score for a patient is obtained by adding the individual scores for each prognostic factor.

- Nongestational choriocarcinoma has a much worse prognosis due to decreased chemosensitivity. Adverse risk factors include stage IV disease or a cumulative risk score >12 in women (Table 7b.3).[16]
- FIGO prognostic score (adapted WHO score):
  - Low risk: <7
  - High risk: ≥7

REFERENCES

1. Lurain JR. Gestational trophoblastic disease I: Epidemiology, pathology, clinical presentation and diagnosis of gestational trophoblastic disease, and management of hydatidiform mole. Am. J. Obstet. Gynecol. 2010; 203:531–9.
2. Salani R, Eisenhauer EL, Copeland LJ. Malignant Diseases and Pregnancy. Obstetrics Normal and Problem Pregnancies. Sixth Edition. Philadelphia: Elsevier; 2012.
3. Brown J, Naumann RW, Seckl MJ et al. 15 years of progress in gestational trophoblastic disease: Scoring, standardization, and salvage. Gynecol Oncol. 2017; 144:200–7.
4. Smith HO, Hilgers RD, Bedrick EJ et al. Ethnic differences at risk for gestational trophoblastic disease in New Mexico: A 25-year population-based study. Am. J. Obstet. Gynecol. 2003; 188(2):357–66.
5. Li AJ. Danforth's Obstetrics and Gynecology. Tenth Edition. Philadelphia: Lippincott Williams & Wilkins; 2008.
6. Cunningham FG. Williams Obstetrics. Twenty-Third Edition. New York: McGraw-Hill Education; 2010.
7. Resnik R, Lockwood CJ, Moore TR, Greene MF, Copel JA, Silver R.M. Creasy and Resnik's Maternal-Fetal Medicine: Principles and Practice. Philadelphia: Elsevier; 2018.
8. Berkowitz RS, Goldstein DP. Molar pregnancy. N Engl J Med. 2009; 360:1639–45.
9. Elias KM, Berkowitz RS, Horowitz NS. State-of-the-art workup and initial management of newly diagnosed molar pregnancy and postmolar gestational trophoblastic neoplasia. J Natl Compr Cancer Netw. 2019; 17:1396–1401.
10. Mutch D, Diver E, Reynolds RK. National Comprehensive Cancer Network (NCCN) Guidelines Version 2.2020 Gestational Trophoblastic Neoplasia [Updated 2020 May 19]. Available from: www.nccn.org [Accessed 2020 Sep 23].
11. Bishop BN, Edemekong PF. Choriocarcinoma [Updated 2020 Jul 14]. StatPearls [Internet]. Treasure Island, FL: StatPearls Publishing. Available from: www.ncbi.nlm.nih.gov/books/NBK535434 [Accessed 2020 Sep 01].
12. DiSaia PJ, Creasman WT, Mannel RS, McMeekin DS, Mutch DG. Clinical

Gynecologic Oncology. Ninth Edition. Philadelphia: Elsevier; 2018.

13. Ulbright M. Germ cell tumors of the gonads: A selective review emphasizing problems in differential diagnosis, newly appreciated, and controversial issues. Mod Pathol. 2005; 18(Suppl 2):S61–79.

14. Barakat RR, Markman M, Randall ME. Principals and Practice of Gynecologic Oncology. Fifth Edition. Baltimore: Lippincott Williams & Wilkins; 2009.

15. Shih IeM. Gestational trophoblastic neoplasia—pathogenesis and potential therapeutic targets. Lancet Oncol. 2007; 8(7):642–50.

16. Lurain JR. Gestational trophoblastic disease II: Classification and management of gestational trophoblastic neoplasia. Am. J. Obstet. Gynecol. 2011; 204(1):11–8.

Polycystic ovarian syndrome, metabolic syndrome, and obesity in pregnancy

LAURA DAVISSON

KEY POINTS

- Polycystic ovarian syndrome (PCOS)
  - PCOS is common in women and characterized by androgen excess, ovulatory dysfunction, and polycystic ovaries.
  - Treatment varies depending on individual patient goals.
  - Many women with PCOS also have metabolic syndrome and obesity which may lead to difficulty conceiving. Weight loss may be pursued to induce ovulation and to aid in successful conception.
  - Certain medications for treatment of PCOS may need to be discontinued when becoming pregnant.
  - Women with PCOS are at risk for gestational diabetes mellitus (GDM) so early screening is recommended.
- Metabolic syndrome
  - This is described as a cluster of abnormalities associated with risk for development of atherosclerotic cardiovascular disease (CVD) and/or type II DM.
  - It is important that patients with metabolic syndrome be identified so that aggressive lifestyle modifications focused on weight management and physical activity can be implemented to reduce the risks of CVD and type II DM.

- Metabolic syndrome is defined by the presence of three of five features, including increased waist circumference, low HDL, high triglycerides, hypertension, and hyperglycemia.
  - Gestational DM and preeclampsia are 2–4 times more likely to occur in pregnant patients with metabolic syndrome.
- Obesity
  - Obesity can decrease the ability to conceive and carries risks during pregnancy; therefore, women should be advised to try to achieve a healthy weight prior to conception.
  - Women with obesity have lower recommended gestational weight gain (GWG) targets than women with normal pre-pregnancy weights but are at risk for gaining more weight than recommended.
  - Women with obesity should be counseled on nutrition, physical activity, and behavior changes to help avoid excessive weight gain during pregnancy.
  - Anti-obesity medications should not be used during pregnancy.
  - There are unique concerns to consider when caring for pregnant women who have had bariatric surgery.

DOI: 10.1201/9781003027577-40

INTRODUCTION

- PCOS, metabolic syndrome, and obesity often coexist and play significant roles in women's reproductive health. PCOS is characterized by androgen excess, ovulatory dysfunction, and polycystic ovaries. Metabolic syndrome is a cluster of metabolic abnormalities associated with the development of CVD and type II DM. Insulin resistance is often noted in these conditions and is associated with skin tags and acanthosis nigricans.
- In women of childbearing age, the prevalence of obesity is 34% and the prevalence of PCOS is 10–18%.[1,2] The prevalence of PCOS is higher in women with overweight and obesity at 28%.[3] Women at high risk for developing PCOS include those with family history, certain ethnicities (Mexican Americans, Australian aborigines), and those who have used antiepileptic drugs, particularly valproate.
- Fifty to eighty percent of women with PCOS have obesity and/or insulin resistance, with the development of DM in more than half by age 40. Women with PCOS also exhibit a higher prevalence of metabolic syndrome.[4]
- Metabolic syndrome prevalence increases with higher weights and is present in 60% of those with obesity. While many people with metabolic syndrome have obesity, it is also possible to see the consequences of metabolic syndrome in some patients without obesity and within certain ethnic groups with lower body mass index (BMI) levels.[5]
- If women take medications for PCOS, metabolic syndrome, or obesity, the safety profile should be evaluated for use during pregnancy.
  - Women should use adequate contraception if drugs are contraindicated during pregnancy, as in the case with spironolactone, statins, and certain anti-hypertensive agents.
  - It is recommended that any non-essential medications be discontinued while trying to conceive and that any medication contraindicated during pregnancy be discontinued, at the latest, upon recognition of conception.
- During pregnancy, a healthy diet and adequate physical activity should generally be continued.
- After pregnancy, breastfeeding should be encouraged in women with PCOS and/or metabolic syndrome, as lactation can improve glucose tolerance and insulin sensitivity, reduce the risk of hypertension and type II DM, and has long-term cardioprotective effects. The benefits are greater in women with longer breastfeeding duration.
- Infants of women with obesity are at increased risk of future obesity development but breastfeeding can reduce this risk.
- Cesarean delivery has been associated with lower breastfeeding rates, so women who have had cesarean sections may need additional lactation support.
- While most medications are compatible with breastfeeding, the LactMed® database can be used as a reference to confirm the safety of specific agents.
- Women who were diagnosed with GDM should be screened for glucose intolerance 2–4 weeks after delivery.
- After pregnancy, women should be encouraged to try to achieve a healthy weight, which usually requires weight loss after delivery. It is recommended that women try to lose pregnancy-related weight gain prior to subsequent pregnancies, and lifelong weight management should be pursued.

POLYCYSTIC OVARIAN SYNDROME IN PREGNANCY

Definition

- PCOS is a common endocrinopathy in women characterized by androgen excess, ovulatory dysfunction, and polycystic ovarian morphology, often accompanied by infertility.
- The syndrome frequently includes symptoms of hirsutism, acne, and male pattern baldness.[2]
- Women with PCOS often present with obesity, insulin resistance, and features of metabolic syndrome in addition to an increased prevalence of endometrial cancer, nonalcoholic fatty liver disease (NAFLD), dyslipidemia, depression, and obstructive sleep apnea.[6]

Diagnosis

- Diagnosis of PCOS is made by using one of three sets of diagnostic criteria: Rotterdam, National Institutes of Health, or Androgen

Excess and PCOS Society. The criteria utilize three features of PCOS in various combinations to confirm the diagnosis:

- Polycystic ovarian morphology, defined by transvaginal ultrasound evidence of increased follicle number and size (not cysts), is one feature included in the diagnostic criteria, but it is not required by any of them.
- Another feature is hyperandrogenism, defined either clinically, biochemically, or both. Clinical hyperandrogenism is the presence of hirsutism, acne, and male pattern balding. Biochemical hyperandrogenism includes elevated levels of androgens including total testosterone and/or DHEA-S.
- Ovulatory dysfunction is typically identified by unpredictable menses that occur at <21-day or >35-day intervals, frequently with <9 menstrual periods per year. Although it has been used by some clinicians, the luteinizing hormone (LH):follicle-stimulating hormone (FSH) ratio has never been a criterion for the diagnosis of PCOS.[2-6]
- The Rotterdam criteria are generally preferred as they are broad and inclusionary. Diagnosis under this method requires two of the three features: Hyperandrogenism, ovulatory dysfunction, or polycystic ovarian morphology. Table 7c.1 compares the diagnostic criteria.[2]
- PCOS is a diagnosis of exclusion.
  - Non-classic congenital adrenal hyperplasia can closely mimic PCOS, so the common form, due to partial 21-hydroxylase deficiency, should be ruled out with an early-morning, early follicular phase plasma 17-hydroxyprogesterone level of less than 200 ng/dL.
  - Pregnancy, hyperprolactinemia, hypothyroidism, primary ovarian insufficiency (evaluated by measuring FSH, LH, estradiol, and possible anti-Mullerian hormone), and hypogonadotropic hypogonadism (functional hypothalamic amenorrhea, evaluated by measuring FSH and LH) should also be ruled out.
  - Androgen-secreting ovarian or adrenal tumors should be considered in patients with abrupt, rapidly progressive, or severe hyperandrogenism.
  - Cushing's syndrome should be considered in women with suggestive clinical features (see Chapter 4d).[2]

Pathophysiology

- PCOS is a complex genetic disorder. A susceptible genotype that is exposed to environmental or acquired factors may lead to hyperandrogenism and eventual PCOS. Ovaries are the predominant source of excess androgens in PCOS, with some secondary production by the adrenal glands. The hypersecretion of ovarian androgens relates to increased pulse frequency of gonadotropin-releasing hormone (GnRH), high LH concentrations, and insufficient FSH secretion.[2]
- Ovarian androgen production is enhanced by insulin resistance and hyperinsulinemia which reduces sex hormone-binding globulin

Table 7c.1 Diagnostic criteria for PCOS

Features of PCOS	NIH criteria	AE PCOS criteria	Rotterdam criteria
Polycystic ovarian morphology[a]	Optional	Optional	Requires 2 of the 3 features
Hyperandrogenism[b]	Required	Required	
Ovulatory dysfunction[c]	Required	Optional	
	Requires both hyperandrogenism and ovulatory dysfunction	Requires hyperandrogenism and one of the other 2 PCOS features	Any 2 of the PCOS features can be used to make the diagnosis

[a] Defined by evidence of increased follicle number and size.
[b] Clinical (hirsutism, acne, male pattern balding) or biochemical (elevated serum androgen levels).
[c] Defined by unpredictable menses that occur at less than 21-day or greater than 35-day intervals.

(SHBG) levels, thereby increasing androgen bioavailability.

- Insulin resistance results in hyperglycemia and increased insulin secretion from pancreatic beta cells. This hyperinsulinemia leads to changes in the skin (acanthosis) and ovary (hyperthecosis) via activation of IGF-1 receptors.
- Obesity worsens insulin resistance and hyperinsulinemia, but it is unclear if obesity is causative, as PCOS may be associated with a greater propensity for obesity and weight gain.[2]

Treatment

- Women with PCOS, many of whom have obesity, may have difficulty conceiving. Therefore, lifestyle changes and weight loss may be pursued to induce ovulation and achieve conception.
- Fertility can be optimized by addressing factors such as glucose, blood pressure, smoking, alcohol, sleep, and mental health. Weight loss of as little as 5–10% can improve menstrual function and fertility.[2,6]
- Spironolactone is commonly used to blunt androgenic effects in women with PCOS. This medication (pregnancy category C) should be discontinued prior to conception due to risk of male fetal feminization.
- Metformin is commonly prescribed in PCOS but is not recommended as a first-line agent for anovulatory infertility. Metformin crosses the placenta to the fetus, and if used in PCOS, should be discontinued by the end of the first trimester.[7]
- Letrozole is now first-line and preferred over clomiphene for ovulation induction in women with PCOS. It may be used with or without the addition of metformin.
- For women who remain anovulatory despite treatment with oral medications, FSH injections or laparoscopic surgery to induce ovulation by destroying androgen-producing cells (ovarian drilling) can be considered.
- In vitro fertilization (IVF) or intracytoplasmic sperm injection (ICSI) may be required. Women with PCOS undergoing IVF +/− ICSI need to be counseled on increased risk of ovarian hyperstimulation syndrome (OHSS).

- Bariatric surgery leads to weight loss and improvement in many of the metabolic effects of PCOS. It improves fertility but is not considered a first-line treatment for infertility in PCOS.[6,8]
- During pregnancy, close monitoring of maternal and fetal health is important given increased risks of adverse maternal and offspring outcomes in women with PCOS including GDM, pregnancy-induced hypertension, preeclampsia, and preterm birth.
  - Oral glucose tolerance test (OGTT) should be offered as screening in all women with PCOS when planning pregnancy or, if currently pregnant, at <20 weeks gestation because of the high risk of hyperglycemia. Women should also have the screening repeated at the usual time of 24–28 weeks gestation.
  - Women with PCOS should be advised to avoid excess gestational weight gain (GWG).[6,9]

METABOLIC SYNDROME IN PREGNANCY

Definition and diagnosis

- Metabolic syndrome is described as a cluster of abnormalities (abdominal obesity, hyperglycemia, dyslipidemia, and hypertension) associated with risk for development of metabolic diseases, primarily CVD and/or type II DM. To reduce these risks, the key clinical implication of the diagnosis is identification of patients who need aggressive lifestyle modifications focused on weight reduction and increased physical activity.
- Patients with metabolic syndrome are at 2-fold risk for developing CVD and at 5-fold risk for developing type II DM.[5] Insulin resistance related to metabolic syndrome has been associated with several metabolic disorders, including NAFLD, hypertension, chronic kidney disease, PCOS, obstructive sleep apnea, and gout. Gestational diabetes and preeclampsia are 2–4 times more likely in metabolic syndrome, and pregnant women with metabolic syndrome have a higher risk for preterm birth.[7,10]

- The 2001 National Cholesterol Education Panel (NCEP) Adult Treatment Panel III (ATP III) criteria for diagnosis of metabolic syndrome is the most widely used definition. Diagnosis requires the presence of three of five features[11]:
  - Abdominal obesity with waist circumference ≥40 inches in men and ≥35 inches in women
  - HDL < 40 mg/dL in men and <50 mg/dL in women
  - Triglycerides ≥ 150 mg/dL
  - Blood pressure ≥ 130/85 mmHg
  - Fasting glucose ≥ 110 mg/dL
- Criteria are also met using drug treatment for any of those conditions.
- Metabolic syndrome is usually identified prior to pregnancy, as diagnosis during pregnancy is complicated by the inability to use waist circumference as one of the diagnostic criteria.
- Risk of metabolic syndrome varies by age, race, weight, postmenopausal status, and household income. Family history and genetics influence risk. Other risk factors include[12–15]:
  - Use of atypical antipsychotic medications, especially clozapine
  - Smoking
  - High carbohydrate diet and sugar-sweetened beverage consumption
  - Lack of alcohol consumption
  - Physical inactivity

Pathophysiology

- The underlying pathophysiology of metabolic syndrome is unclear, which contributes to uncertainty about the diagnosis.
- Many factors other than metabolic syndrome affect the likelihood that a person with obesity will develop DM or CVD, including genetic predisposition, lack of exercise, and body fat distribution.
- Obesity is associated with decreased adiponectin.
- Adiponectin, secreted by adipose tissue, has the protective effects of being insulin-sensitizing, anti-atherogenic, and anti-inflammatory. Decreased levels can lead to high circulating levels of insulin and triglycerides, hypertension, and vascular inflammation, all of which promote the development of atherosclerotic CVD in genetically predisposed individuals.[16]

Treatment

- Healthy diet, exercise, and weight management are the only recommended interventions for metabolic syndrome. Treatment also involves managing the components of the syndrome and the cardiovascular risk factors of smoking, hypertension, hyperglycemia, and hyperlipidemia. Any medications being used for those conditions which are contraindicated in pregnancy should be discontinued, if possible, upon recognition of conception.

OBESITY IN PREGNANCY

Definition and diagnosis

- The diagnosis of obesity in the non-pregnant population is most commonly based on a BMI of ≥30 kg/m². An alternative diagnosis consists of waist circumference >40 inches in men or >35 inches in women.
- There are several obesity classes: class 1 (BMI 30+), class 2 (BMI 35+), and class 3 (BMI 40+).
- Since weight gain in pregnancy often begins before the first prenatal visit and with inability to utilize waist circumference, diagnosis of obesity in pregnancy is based on pre-pregnancy weight. Prepregnancy weight is more strongly associated with adverse maternal and infant outcomes than GWG.[17]
- Obesity is associated with DM, hypertension, obstructive sleep apnea, CVD, metabolic syndrome, PCOS, NAFLD, and endometrial cancer.
- Obesity in pregnancy is associated with multiple adverse conditions:
  - Early pregnancy loss
  - Gestational DM
  - Pregnancy-associated hypertension
  - Preeclampsia
  - Preterm birth
  - Post-term pregnancy
  - Cesarean delivery
  - Macrosomia
  - Venous thromboembolism
  - Infection
  - Postpartum depression
  - Congenital anomalies
  - Fetal death
  - Large-for-gestational-age infants

- Postpartum weight retention and worsening obesity
- Maternal morbidity increases with higher obesity classes. Adverse outcomes include cardiac and respiratory morbidity, shock, and a combined outcome of "severe maternal morbidity or mortality."[18-20]

Pathophysiology

- Etiology of obesity is multifactorial, including genetics, hormonal abnormalities, diet, physical activity, stress, and psychological factors, the food environment, sleep, medications, and socioeconomic status.
- Obesity may result in pathogenic adipose tissue that contributes to metabolic disease, which develops when positive caloric balance in genetically and environmentally susceptible individuals results in adverse clinical consequences (metabolic diseases).
- Obesity is associated with insulin resistance and increased risk of development of type II DM.
- The offspring of women who have obesity during pregnancy are at increased risk of childhood and adult obesity due to epigenetic changes induced by fetal exposure to increased levels of glucose, insulin, lipids, and inflammatory cytokines.
- Shared familial lifestyle also plays a role in the increased risk of obesity in offspring.[21]

Treatment

- Obesity is associated with decreased fertility. Weight loss can be helpful for improving fertility. Women should be educated on the benefits of achieving healthy weight prior to pregnancy.
- Institute of Medicine (IOM) 2009 guidelines recommend that all women should strive to be within the normal BMI range when they conceive. This should be included in preconception counseling, in addition to other standard preconception recommendations.[1]
- As little as 10% weight loss prior to conception may reduce risks associated with obesity including preeclampsia, GDM, preterm delivery, macrosomia, and stillbirth.[20]
- Medical professionals should offer evidence-based tools to help patients with weight management prior to conception and between pregnancies.
- While all women should be screened for GDM with an OGTT at 24–28 weeks, this should be performed earlier in women with obesity where there is a higher degree of suspicion for DM.
- Ultrasound screenings may be more difficult to obtain in pregnant women with obesity, and techniques may need to be adjusted. Transvaginal sonography may offer improved ascertainment of nuchal translucency measurements. Neural tube and other defects may also be challenging to assess by ultrasound. Obstetrical ultrasound assessment of the fetal heart may be suboptimal. Women should be counseled about the limitations of these tests. Alternative screenings such as a maternal serum α-fetoprotein or a fetal echo can be considered, although they are not routinely indicated.[20]
- Diagnostic procedures including amniocentesis and chorionic villus sampling are more technically challenging in pregnant women with obesity and special techniques may be needed to improve success rates.
- In the third trimester, assessment of fetal growth by abdominal palpation and fundal height measurement may be challenging in women with obesity, so it may be useful to consider assessing fetal growth with ultrasound every 4–6 weeks.
- Some experts recommend delivery by the estimated due date to reduce the risk of stillborn birth, but this is controversial.[22]
- During labor, there are several considerations for women with obesity.
  - Labor and delivery units should be prepared with the proper equipment and gowns to accommodate patients of any size.
  - Fetal monitoring with external Doppler ultrasound transducers may be difficult to use, so monitoring may require internal fetal scalp electrodes.
  - There may also be higher risks for anesthesia complications in patients with obesity.[20]

WEIGHT GAIN DURING PREGNANCY

- Preventing excessive weight gain during pregnancy is important, as women with obesity are

Table 7c.2 Institute of Medicine (IOM) 2009 Gestational weight targets for singleton pregnancy

Pre-pregnancy BMI (kg/m²)	Recommended pregnancy weight gain (kg)
<18.5	12.5–18
18.5–24.9	11.5–16
25–29.9	7–11.5
30+	5–9

at increased risk for excessive GWG, which has negative health effects on both the mother and infant. However, inadequate GWG carries risk of delivery of a small for gestational age (SGA) newborn.

- Weight loss while pregnant is associated with adverse outcomes and should not be encouraged. Anti-obesity medications should not be used during pregnancy.
- Pregnant women with obesity have lower recommended GWG targets than women with normal prepregnancy weights but are at risk for gaining more weight than recommended (see Table 7c.2). Targets on the lower end of the range are recommended for women with class 2 or 3 obesity.[1,23]
- Only a minority of women surveyed report being counseled correctly about how much weight to gain during pregnancy or about the risks of inappropriate weight gain.[24] A survey of obstetric providers noted that 37% did not know the minimum BMI for diagnosing obesity and most advised GWGs that were discordant with IOM guidelines in effect at that time.[17]
- Women with obesity should be counseled on nutrition, physical activity, and behavior changes to help avoid excessive weight gain during pregnancy.
  - Lifestyle interventions can prevent excessive GWG by 20%.[1,25]
  - Women should be advised that caloric intake does not need to increase until the second and third trimesters, and they need only increase by 300 kcals per day to gain 1 lb/week. For women with obesity, even less of a caloric increase is needed.
  - Pregnant women can safely continue most pre-pregnancy exercise programs or even initiate new physical activity programs as

this may improve pregnancy outcomes. Exercise may help to prevent excessive weight gain, although a meta-analysis of interventions done to optimize GWG concluded that focusing on exercise may be lower yield than focusing on nutrition.[1]

BARIATRIC SURGERY CONSIDERATIONS

- Fertility increases after bariatric surgery due to reduced insulin resistance, decreased androgen levels, and return of ovulation. The return of fertility can be rapid, with oligomenorrheic women reporting resuming normal menstrual cycles 3.4 months postoperatively.
- Many women do not recognize how easily they may become pregnant after bariatric surgery and they should be counseled to use contraception if they do not want to conceive. Women who have had bariatric surgery should consider the use of an IUD or other nonoral method for contraception after pregnancy given possibility of malabsorption with oral medications.
- Experts recommend delaying pregnancy for 12–24 months after bariatric surgery to allow for optimization of weight loss and reduce potentially adverse effects of nutrient deficiency on neonatal outcomes.[26]
- Potential harms of prepregnancy bariatric surgery include:
  - Small-for-gestational-age fetus
  - Premature delivery
  - Possibly increased infant mortality
- Potential benefits include reduced incidence of:
  - Large-for-gestational-age fetus
  - Gestational DM
  - Hypertensive disorders of pregnancy
- Women who have had bariatric surgery have higher cesarean section rates than the general obstetric population but similar or lower rates compared to women with obesity who have not undergone bariatric surgery.[6,26]
- Optimal weight gain during pregnancy in women who have previously undergone bariatric surgery has not been studied; thus, current recommendations are based on IOM guidelines and pre-pregnancy BMI.
- Serial ultrasounds are often done every 4 weeks to evaluate fetal growth in the third trimester, especially if there is poor weight gain or if the woman conceived within two years of bariatric surgery.

- Bariatric surgeries can be classified into either restrictive (e.g., adjustable laparoscopic band (lap band), sleeve gastrectomy) or malabsorptive (e.g., Roux-en-Y gastric bypass, biliopancreatic diversion with duodenal switch). More nutrient deficiencies are seen after malabsorptive surgeries and medication absorption may also be impaired.
- To prevent deficiencies due to weight loss and malabsorption, vitamin supplementation is routinely prescribed after bariatric surgery. Pregnant women who have had bariatric surgery should continue the supplements they were taking prior to pregnancy except they should replace the multivitamin with a prenatal vitamin. Depending on the supplement, additional iron and folate may be required. Patients should not receive more than 5000 IUs of vitamin A to avoid retinoid embryopathy.
- Pregnant women who have had bariatric surgery should be screened for nutrient deficiencies as early as possible and every trimester so that supplementation regimens can be tailored to the individual patient. Laboratory tests include:
  - Complete blood count (CBC)
  - Ferritin
  - Iron
  - Vitamin B12
  - Thiamine
  - Folate
  - Calcium
  - Vitamin D
- Any deficiency should be corrected and monitored monthly.
- If iron replacement is needed, intravenous supplementation is generally preferred over oral to ensure adequate replacement and avoid gastrointestinal toxicities. If given orally, iron should be dosed daily or every other day.[26]
- Wernicke's encephalopathy from thiamine deficiency may be a concern if a woman with a history of gastric bypass surgery has hyperemesis.
- Patients with a history of bariatric surgery should be counseled to report abdominal pain to their healthcare provider. Gallstones are common during periods of rapid weight loss and have increased prevalence in pregnancy. Bowel obstruction is a rare late sequela of bariatric surgery. There is also a risk of gastric ulceration after bariatric surgery and therefore, in the postpartum period, use of nonsteroidal anti-inflammatory drugs (NSAIDs) for postpartum pain should be avoided.
- Lactation is not adversely affected by bariatric surgery and should be encouraged, although babies who are exclusively breastfed from women who have had gastric bypass surgery may develop deficiencies if maternal nutrient deficiency monitoring is not continued.
- Breastfeeding women who have had bariatric surgery should continue to follow supplementation guidelines.

WEIGHT MANAGEMENT IN PCOS, METABOLIC SYNDROME, AND OBESITY

- Pregnant women with PCOS, metabolic syndrome, and/or obesity should follow the basic principles of a high quality, whole food diet. The diet choice can be individualized based on personal factors and food preferences.[6]
- Weight regain is common if the patient returns to a former eating pattern that initially led to weight gain.
- Physical activity should be encouraged. In addition to the benefits of exercise on weight loss, exercise may also be beneficial for abdominal adiposity and reduction of CVD risk.
- The main benefit of exercise regarding weight management specifically is in maintenance rather than weight loss, which is more influenced by food intake.
- Behavioral strategies that assist with lifestyle modification adherence include goal-setting, self-monitoring, and stimulus control (controlling the food environment).[21]
- Other factors to assist with weight management include adequate sleep, limiting weight-promoting medications, and managing psychological factors that can affect weight.
- Regardless of the strategy used to achieve optimal weight, weight management outcomes are improved when patients have frequent follow-up appointments, preferably at least monthly.[21,27]
- Anti-obesity medications are contraindicated in pregnancy but may be used prior to pregnancy or postpartum.[6] When used in the postpartum period, available options are reviewed in Table 7c.3.[27]

Table 7c.3 Anti-obesity medications approved for long-term use

Medication	Dosing	Main contraindications[a]
Phentermine-Topiramate (Schedule IV)	Starter pack: 3.75/23 mg daily for 14 days then 7.5/46 mg daily; max 15/92 mg daily	Heart disease, kidney stones
Bupropion-Naltrexone 8/90 mg	Start 1 tablet daily for 1 week, then 1 tablet twice a day for 1 week, then 2 tablets in the morning and 1 tablet at night for 1 week, then 2 tablets twice daily	Seizure disorder, active use of narcotics
Liraglutide	Start at 0.6 mg subcutaneous injection daily, increase by 0.6 mg increments weekly to max of 3 mg daily	Pancreatitis, personal or family history of medullary thyroid cancer or MEN syndrome
Semaglutide	Start at 0.25 mg subcutaneous injection weekly × 4 weeks then 0.5 mg weekly × 4 weeks then 1 mg weekly × 4 weeks then 1.7 mg weekly × 4 weeks then 2.4 mg weekly	Pancreatitis, personal or family history of medullary thyroid cancer or MEN syndrome

[a] Pregnancy is a contraindication to any anti-obesity medication.

- Bariatric surgery may be performed postpartum. If bariatric surgery is considered prior to conception, pregnancy should be delayed for 12–24 months postoperatively.

REFERENCES

1. Craemer, KA, E Sampene, N Safdar, KM Antony, and CK Wautlet. 2019. "Nutrition and Exercise Strategies to Prevent Excessive Pregnancy Weight Gain: A meta-analysis Nutrition and Exercise." *AJP Reports* 9 (1): e92–e120.
2. McCartney, C. 2016. "Polycystic Ovary Syndrome." *NEJM* 375: 54–64.
3. Alvarez-Blasco, F, B Botella-Carretero, JL San Millan, and HF Escobar-Morreale. 2006. "Prevalence and Characteristics of the Polycystic Ovary Syndrome in Overweight and Obese Women." *Archives of Internal Medicine* 166: 2081–2086.
4. Chandrasekaran, S, and H Sagili. 2018. "Metabolic Syndrome in Women with Polycystic Ovary Syndrome." *The Obstetrician & Gynaecologist* 20: 245–252.
5. Kip, KE, OC Marroquin, DE Kelley, and BD Johnson. 2004. "Clinical Importance of Obesity Versus the Metabolic Syndrome in Cardiovascular Risk in Women: A Report From the Women's Ischemia Syndrome Evaluation (WISE) Study." *Circulation* 109(6): 706–713.
6. Teede, HJ, ML Misso, MF Costello, A Dokras, J Laven, L Moran, T Piltonen, RJ Norman, and International PCOS Network. 2018. "Recommendations from the International Evidence-Based Guideline for the Assessment and Management of Polycystic Ovary Syndrome." *Fertility and Sterility* 110 (3): 364–379.
7. American Diabetes Association. 2020. "Standards of Medical Care in Diabetes—2020 Abridged for Primary Care Providers." *Clinical Diabetes* 38 (1): 10–38.
8. Gadalla, MA, RJ Norman, CT Tay, DS Hiam, A Melder, J Pundir, S Thangaratinam, HJ Teede, BW Mol, and LJ Moran. 2020. "Medical and Surgical Treatment of Reproductive Outcomes in Polycystic Ovary Syndrome: An Overview of Systematic Reviews." *International Journal of Fertility and Sterility* 13 (4): 257–270.
9. Zheng, W, W Huang, L Zhang, Z Tian, Q Yan, T Wang, L Zhang, and G Li. 2019. "Early Pregnancy Metabolic Factors Associated with Gestational Diabetes Mellitus in Normal-Weight Women with Polycystic Ovary Syndrome: A Two-Phase Cohort Study." *Diabetology & Metabolic Syndrome* 11(71): 1–9.

10. Chatzi, L, E Plana, V Daraki, P Karakosta, D Alegkakis, C Tsatsanis, A Kafatos, A Koutis, and M Kogevinas. 2009. "Metabolic Syndrome in Early Pregnancy and Risk of Preterm Birth." *American Journal of Epidemiology* 170 (7): 829–836.

11. Expert Panel on Detection, Evaluation, and Treatment of High Blood Cholesterol in Adults. 2001. "Executive Summary of the Third Report of the National Cholesterol Education Program (NCEP) Expert Panel on Detection, Evaluation, and Treatment of High Blood Cholesterol in Adults." *JAMA* 285(19): 2486–2497.

12. Park, YW, Zhu S, and Palaniappan L. 2003. "The Metabolic Syndrome: Prevalence and Associated Risk Factor Findings in the US Population from the Third National Health and Nutrition Examination Survey." *Archives of Internal Medicine 163(4)*: 427–436.

13. Carnethon, MR, CM Loria, JO Hill, S Sidney, PJ Savage, and K Liu. 2004. "Risk Factors for the Metabolic Syndrome. The Coronary Artery Risk Development in Young Adults (CARDIA) Study, 1985–2001." *Diabetes Care.* 27(11): 2707–2715.

14. Al-Qawasmeh, R, and R Tayyem. 2018. "Dietary and Lifestyle Risk Factors and Metabolic Syndrome: Literature Review." *Current Research in Nutrition and Food Science.* 6(3): 594–608.

15. Lamberti, JS, D Olson, JF Crilly, T Olivares, GC Williams, X Tu, W Tang, K Wiener, S Dvorin, and MB Dietz. 2006. "Prevalence of the Metabolic Syndrome Among Patients Receiving Clozapine." *American Journal of Psychiatry.* 163(7): 1273–1276.

16. Grundy, SM, HB Brewer, JI Cleeman, SC Smith, and C Lenfant. 2004. "Definition of Metabolic Syndrome." *Circulation.* 109(3): 433–438.

17. Herring, S, DN Platek, P Elliott, and LE Riley. 2010. "Addressing Obesity in Pregnancy: What Do Obstetric Providers Recommend?" *Journal of Women's Health* 19 (1): 65–70.

18. Lisonkova, S, GM Muraca, J Potts, J Liauw, WS Chan, A Skoll, and KI Lim. 2017. "Association Between Prepregnancy Body Mass Index and Severe Maternal Morbidity." *JAMA.* 318(18): 1777–1786.

19. Stubert, J, F Reister, S Hartmann, and W Janni. 2018. "The Risks Associated with Obesity in Pregnancy." *Deutsches Ärzteblatt International.* 115(16): 276–283.

20. American College of Obstetrics and Gynecologists. 2015. "Practice Bulletin No. 156 Obesity in Pregnancy." *Obstetrics & Gynecology* 126(6): e112–126.

21. Bays, HE, W McCarthy, S Christensen, J Tondt, S Karjoo, L Davisson, J Ng et al. 2020. *Obesity Algorithm eBook.* www.obesityalgorithm.org.

22. Denison, FC, NR Aedla, O Keag, K Hor, RM Reynolds, A Milne, and A Diamond. 2018. "Care of Women with Obesity in Pregnancy. Green-top Guideline No. 72." *BJOG.* 126(3): e62–e106.

23. Rasmussen KM, AL Yaktine, Institute of Medicine (US) and National Research Council (US) Committee to Reexamine IOM Pregnancy Weight Guidelines, eds. *Weight Gain During Pregnancy: Reexamining the Guidelines.* Washington (DC): National Academies Press (US); 2009.

24. McDonald, SD, E Pullenayegum, VH Taylor, E Pullenayegum, O Lutsiv, K Bracken, C Good, E Hutton, and W. Sword. 2011. "Despite 2009 Guidelines, Few Women Report Being Counseled Correctly About Weight Gain During Pregnancy." *American Journal of Obstetrics and Gynecology.* (6): CD007145.

25. Muktabhant, B, TA Lawrie, P Lumbiganon, and M Laopaiboon. 2015. "Diet or Exercise, or Both, for Preventing Excessive Weight Gain in Pregnancy." *Cochrane Database of Systematic Reviews* 205(4): 333.e1–6

26. Kominiarek, MA. 2011. "Preparing for and Managing a Pregnancy After Bariatric Surgery." *Semin Perinatol.* 35(6): 356–361.

27. Apovian, CM, LJ Arrone, DH Bessesen, ME McDonnell, H Murad, U Pagotto, DH Ryan, and CD Still. 2015. "Pharmacological Management of Obesity: An Endocrine Society Clinical Practice Guideline." *Journal of Clinical Endocrinology & Metabolism.* 100(2): 342–362.

Index